Language Sample Analysis:
The Wisconsin Guide

Barbara J. Leadholm
Consultant, Speech and Language Handicapped Programs
Bureau for Exceptional Children

Jon F. Miller
Professor, University of Wisconsin-Madison
Waisman Center on Mental Retardation
and Human Development

Wisconsin Department of Public Instruction
Madison, Wisconsin

This publication is available from:

Publication Sales
Wisconsin Department of Public Instruction
Drawer 179
Milwaukee, WI 53293-0179
(800) 243-8782

Bulletin No. 92424

Reviewed and Approved for Reprint January 1995

© 1992 Wisconsin Department of Public Instruction

ISBN 1-57337-011-8

Printed on
Recycled Paper

Contents of the Guide

Wisconsin has long been a leader in the field of education. It is a state committed to providing *all* students a free, appropriate public education. In order to meet that commitment, we, as educators, must be diligent in our efforts to continually monitor our methods of evaluation, intervention strategies, and programs developed for students with identified exceptional educational needs.

This publication (along with follow-up training) has been developed as a result of that commitment. For many years, speech and language pathologists and directors of special education have been requesting more specific guidance to assist them in identifying students with oral communication disabilities.

It is anticipated that the information presented in this publication about language sample analysis (LSA) and data collected in Wisconsin over the past nine years will increase the utilization, consistency, and reliability of language sampling for children in the state with suspected or identified language production disabilities. It will also provide a detailed description of language performance from which a specific intervention plan can be developed. This information is also a great help in effectively monitoring the specific progress of children receiving intervention.

I encourage you to expand your knowledge and use of language sample analysis. The cost effective technologies described within this publication will provide greater consistency in the identification of children with expressive language disabilities among speech and language pathologists within Wisconsin school districts.

John T. Benson
State Superintendent

Acknowledgments

The Wisconsin Department of Public Instruction gratefully acknowledges the contributions of a number of dedicated people who have given their valuable time, talent, and expertise to the development of this publication. Thanks and appreciation is also due their local school districts for allowing participation on this task force, despite other pressing district responsibilities. Our thanks go to the following individuals involved in the development of this publication:

Christine Freiberg
Speech/Language Pathologist
Wausau School District
Wausau

Surita Hall-Smith
Supervisor of Speech/Language
  and Hearing Impaired Programs
Green Bay Area School District
Green Bay

Pat Johnson
Elementary Principal
K-12 Curriculum Coordinator
Johnson Creek School District
Johnson Creek

Barbara Rademaker
Speech/Language Pathologist
Mosinee School District
Mosinee

Teresa Goodier
Speech/Language Pathologist
Program Support Teacher
CESA 10
Chippewa Falls

Jim Larson
Director of Special Education
CESA 9
Tomahawk

Kathleen Lyngaas
Speech/Language Pathologist
Program Support Teacher
Madison Metropolitan School District
Madison

Teri Mills
District Administrator
Lodi School District
Lodi

Carol Schmidt
Speech/Language Disabilities
Program Supervisor
Milwaukee Public Schools
Milwaukee

Special recognition and thanks goes to:

Dr. Brent Zimmerman, Business Manager, Mosinee, for his diligence in keeping our project fiscally sound.

The Speech and Language Pathologists from the Madison Metropolitan School District and CESA 9, without whose work in LSA this publication would not be possible.

Department of Public Instruction staff to be thanked are Margaret T. Dwyer, text editor; Victoria Rettenmund, graphic artist, Dianne Penman, management information technician; Hazel Fedro, word processing operator, Lisa Isgitt and Jessica Early, proofreaders.

Introduction

Language sample analysis (LSA) has long been considered as one of the best evaluative procedures of expressive language performance. Several factors, however, have limited its general use including a lack of standardized procedures for eliciting language samples, validated measurement categories, normative data, and relevant interpretation strategies. Over the past several years, each of these issues has received attention from funded research projects conducted in Wisconsin's public schools. The results have led to the development of standardized language sampling procedures, language sample norms, and interpretation strategies, all of which can be used in the evaluation process for determining the existence of a handicapping condition in expressive language production. The resulting data also have direct implications for determining special education program intervention strategies, and in monitoring student progress.

The goal of this publication is to share information about Language Sample Analysis (LSA) and to explain

- *why* it is critical to the appropriate evaluation of students;
- *who* it should benefit;
- *how* it can be accomplished; and
- *what* information it will provide.

The development of this guide was motivated by several issues: the continued statewide increase in speech and language prevalence rates; requests from speech and language pathologists (SLPs) to provide guidelines which will assist in the appropriate determination of a handicapping condition; and a need for statewide norms of expressive language production. When the Madison Metropolitan School District (MMSD) SLPs first met in 1982 to consider how they could effectively implement LSA in a school environment, they identified two goals as central to success. The first was the establishment of a standard method of collecting, recording, transcribing, and analyzing language samples. The second was the need for a referenced database of typically developing school-age children that would lead to consistent interpretation of test results. This group of SLPs met the first goal when they developed a functional approach to collection, transcription, and analysis of language samples.

Meeting the second goal was more difficult because it required the collection of language samples of typically developing children in standard speaking conditions. This project was undertaken in 1984 by the MMSD and the Language Analysis Laboratory of the University of Wisconsin-Madison. The result has been the development of the Reference Database (RDB), a set of criterion referenced measures of language performance for children three to 13 years of age. The Madison sample contained 192 children, three, four, five, six, seven, nine, 11, and 13 years of age, with 27 to 30 children in each group. Application of the RDB statewide raised issues regarding the representativeness of the Madison children, particularly rural populations. To evaluate this question, CESA-9 and the Language Analysis Lab in 1987 collected samples from 90 children from rural north-central Wisconsin, 30 each at three, five, and seven years of age. Comparison of these samples with the MMSD data revealed no significant statistical differences between them on developmental measures of language performance. The RDB, which combines both of these data sets, can be found in Appendix A. The combined total of students in the RDB is 266.

This guide extends the use of Language Sample Analysis in school settings in three important ways. First, it provides a standard methodology for conducting LSA in school settings; second, it includes a set of data derived from Wisconsin children to aid speech and language pathologists' interpretations of language sample analysis; and third, it categorizes different types of productive language impairment developed by school-based speech and language pathologists.

Section 1 provides an overview of the language sampling analysis process and types of language disorders while Section 2 discusses the sampling process in detail. Section 3 describes the transcription process and coding conventions; Section 4 describes analytical procedures that cover various aspects of productive language. A step-by-step review of a case study is included in Section 5 to assist in the interpretation of data provided by the RDB as well as the development of intervention plans for the child's Individualized Education Program (IEP). Section 6 reviews the issues and concerns in documenting language disorders in linguistically and culturally diverse populations as well as in children with cognitive, sensory, or motor deficits. Finally, Section 7 explains how language sample analysis applies to the M-team process.

Appendix A includes the Reference Database. Transcript entry conventions for computer and hand analysis procedures make up Appendixes B and C. Appendix D contains additional resources for further information on LSA and related topics. A glossary of terms used in this guide can be found in Appendix E. Appendix F contains information on the cost-effectiveness of LSA that might be of interest to administrators. Appendix G has sample case studies that SLPs can use to assess different kinds of language problems. Finally, Appendix H contains material on how to meet the needs of linguistically and culturally diverse children (LCD).

A basic level of training in the principles and assumptions underlying language sample analysis is assumed. This guide is meant to augment existing knowledge and experience in assessing productive language using Language Sample Analysis techniques.

Training materials developed by the Department of Public Instruction will be provided following the publication of this document to help further facilitate the dissemination of this material and provide the "hands on" training needed for implementation.

The Need for Language Sample Analysis

Purpose

The purpose of Language Sample Analysis (LSA) is to

- identify or document a language disorder.
- provide the descriptive detail necessary to initiate a focused intervention program.
- provide a method for monitoring progress in language intervention.

Language Sample Analysis uses a recorded and transcribed sample of dialogue between two speakers to identify and describe productive language disorders in school-aged children. LSA is a standardized, quantitative method that evaluates productive language at all levels of performance: vocabulary, syntax, semantics, and pragmatics. The general definitions of these levels apply. Vocabulary refers to the words that a child selects in order to express ideas. Syntax reflects a child's knowledge of English grammar. Semantics indicate the meanings expressed by individual words and sentences. Finally, pragmatics refers to a child's social use of language, communicating ideas, information, needs, and requests.

LSA has four basic components:

- a *sample* of a child's conversation and narration,
- a *transcription* of the recorded language sample,
- an *analysis* of the child's vocabulary, syntax, and semantic and pragmatic features, and
- an *interpretation* of the analysis.

Together, these four components offer a measurement tool that will document a student's oral language proficiency relative to age-matched peers.

Language and the Educational Process

The development of language and communication skills is fundamental for educational progress. Upon school entry, oral language skills are a primary means of acquiring and sharing new information while simultaneously developing advanced language skills in the following: social conventions, grammatical structure, and vocabulary. Through the middle elementary school years, the medium of learning shifts from oral language to reading and writing. Reading skills give students access to new information and writing skills enable students to share this new knowledge with the literate world. By the time students enter their middle and high school years they require appropriate reading and writing skills in order to have access to the educational curriculum. Clearly, early deficits in oral language skills may lead to severe problems with the acquisition of necessary reading and writing skills and can interfere with a student's overall abilities in school.

In Wisconsin's classrooms today, deficits in oral language are the result of diverse factors. Perceptual and cognitive deficits (which include injuries to the central nervous system), emotional problems, environmental influences, and unknown reasons draw educators into the complex puzzle of language problems. School is a language-intensive environment where children engage in language-learning activities on various skill levels and where deficient oral language skills, regardless of the cause, will hinder the educational process. Many children come from environments where print surrounds them, and they quickly find meaning and feel comfortable reading, writing, and spelling; however, some children enter school from environments where print is undervalued or unavailable. Even in today's society, many adults practice the belief that "children should be seen and not heard." Whether voices are actually silenced or just lost in the melee of today's busy world, this silence creates a void that restricts a student's practical use of language in both written and oral form, and impairs language competency. For these children, a mismatch between abilities and curricular demands occurs, and typical language arts activities such as rhyming games, word families, or vocabulary-building activities which require word definitions are difficult. Moreover, as children with poor oral language skills get older, the gap widens: these children are ill-equipped to deal with the vocational and social contexts of language used in adult life. It is little wonder that schools identify children with poorly developed language systems as "at risk" during their first school years.

Each of the modes used in communication to express language—listening, speaking, reading, and writing—are all interrelated and mutually influential. Progress in reading and writing is irretrievably linked to progress in oral language. Currently, whole language is a model of instruction in education that views language as an integrated system which develops through complex interactions from early childhood. In this model, the child's oral language is the foundation for building literacy. Children learn about reading and writing as they talk and listen. They learn about reading as they explore writing, and their oral language improves as they read and write. Such a view of teaching literacy by focusing on meaning and the child's experiences rather than on specific skills parallels current beliefs about how oral language develops. The ongoing challenge is to design assessment and intervention strategies that meet individual student needs, while remaining consistent with knowledge and beliefs.

Because LSA contributes significantly to assessment and intervention strategies, it is vital that speech and language pathologists (SLPs) in Wisconsin obtain and use this consistent methodology and the database. Before relating the specifics of how to sample, transcribe, analyze, and interpret a language sample, it is necessary to review a definition of a language disorder and to present six types of expressive language disorders seen in the caseloads of Wisconsin SLPs.

What Constitutes a Language Disorder?

A language disorder, as the term will be used in this guide, is impaired oral performance that significantly interferes with educational success and appropriate social interaction. In general, language-disordered children show a later onset of language skills, their rate of acquisition is slower, and they may never have the skills of their peers even as adults. (Aram, Ekelman, and Nation, 1984; Schery, 1985; Weiner, 1985)

The term *language disorder* will be used to refer to all types of productive language impairment, where expressive performance significantly deviates from age expectations. *Language delay* refers to one type of language disorder documented by language test results that correlate highly with age. The developmental progress of children with language delay is significantly slower than age peers, but follows the normal sequence of development.

LSA and Disordered Language Performance

Identifying language disorders requires comparing performance on measures of language production with measures of language comprehension, non-verbal abilities, and chronological age. These measures can be compared using a developmental profile. (Miller,

1978; 1981) Figure 1 displays the developmental profiles of three children: child A with language comprehension and production delayed relative to non-verbal cognitive abilities; child B with language production delayed relative to language comprehension and non-verbal cognitive abilities; and child C whose language is developing normally, and language production and comprehension are equal to non-verbal cognitive status and chronological age.

 Figure 1

Developmental Profile

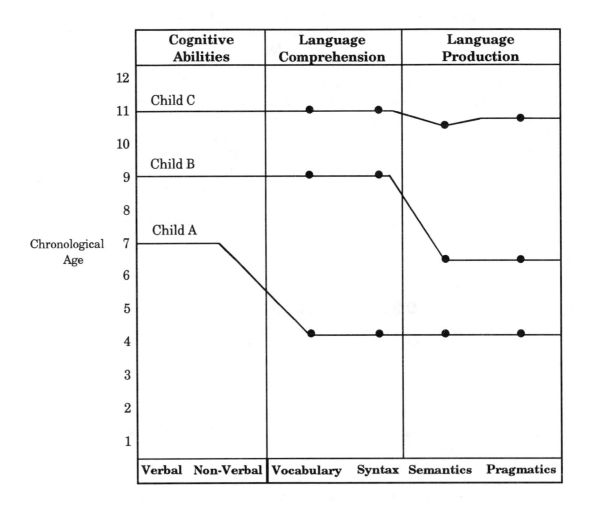

Child A and B exhibit disordered language, but each has a different developmental profile. Note that both of these examples have deficits in language production. The developing demographics of language disorder suggests that production deficits are by far the most frequent, whether they are accompanied by comprehension deficits or not. This profile analysis defines normal development as synchronous cognitive ability, language comprehensions, and language production skills. Language disorder is defined by significant

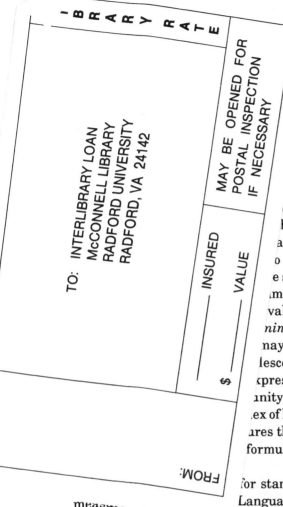

, language comprehension, and cognitive perfor-
ing children chronological age (CA) and cognitive
nilar.

are children who perform well on tests of specific
theless are unable to use language for effective oral
ibit a variety of behaviors that interfere with verbal
duction deficits are difficult to identify with tests of
ese children requires more precise quantification of
se level of analysis.

t integrates the different parts of language with one
h the communication requirements in the student's life
ation problems go undetected in standardized measures
o document. Assessment strategies that isolate discrete
e student's true ability to use language in everyday social
mple, standardized tests such as the Northwest Syntax
valuation of Language Functions (CELF) use repetition of
niner to demonstrate knowledge of syntax. Expressive
nay be measured by a student's ability to use the word in a
lescent Language (TOAL) or by identifying the name of an
xpressive One Word Picture Vocabulary Test. On the other
inity to evaluate through actual conversation and narration.
ex of language performance available to speech and language
ires the development and accuracy of grammatical morphol-
formulation, and discourse in a variety of communication

for standardized language tests but should augment existing
measu... Language evaluations of children should incorporate a variety
of strategies to quantify language comprehension, production, and processing skills. LSA
can be used to validate and expand upon production deficits noted by standardized tests.

However, there are children who exhibit deficits in oral communication skills that
perform within normal limits on tests of language performance. These children represent
a paradox for current identification practice which suggests that if the standardized tests
do not document a language disorder, the child does not have one. For example, teachers
might note oral language deficits relative to peers in the classroom, however language tests
do not confirm the teacher's view. LSA provides a method for quantifying the language
deficits observed by the classroom teacher and SLP. With the methods and performance
data provided by this guide, a more appropriate view of the child's ability to use language
for communication will be obtained.

Finally, standardized tests are often biased and may over-identify or under-identify
disordered language performance; for example, children who come from linguistically and
culturally diverse (LCD) backgrounds that differ from those of children included in the
standardization sample. Even if the standardized test includes the proper representation
of LCD children in the normative sample, educators interpret the results relative to the
mainstream culture. This perspective always places the LCD child at risk for an accurate
evaluation of language and communication ability unless the SLP takes care to differentiate a language disorder from a language difference. Evaluation of the child's
language performance must be done in the context of individual ethnic culture as well as

the culture of the school. Other populations for whom standardized measures of language ability will over- or under-identify include children with attention deficit disorders, children with high test anxiety, and children with short term memory or other information processing disorders. LSA provides the only direct method of approaching these difficult tasks because it measures spontaneous discourse. Solving the assessment problem for the individual child requires that careful attention be paid to identifying valid sampling conditions and cautious use of data for interpretation, particularly where data are primarily from European-American children of the mainstream culture. Some of these issues will be discussed in more detail in Section 6. Resources have been identified for reference and they can be found in Appendix D.

Description

The data from the LSA describes explicitly the deficits that the intervention program will address. Because LSA is based on functional use of language in natural communication contexts, intervention plans can more easily incorporate instruction that will assist the child in academic and social settings. LSA allows the pathologist to probe easy and difficult communication contexts and provides insight into the strategies students may use to solve communication difficulties.

Monitoring Progress

Language Sample Analysis effectively monitors productive language status of children because it measures performance in a variety of everyday speaking situations. It also documents progress for the annual Individualized Education Program (IEP) of children receiving services. In the context of real speaking and listening situations, LSA reveals performance changes that reflect the results of direct instruction and generalization. SLPs can further evaluate generalization's effects by collecting samples of the child's conversation with peers or teacher and in new speaking conditions relevant to the child's curriculum. Just as letter/sound correspondence drill does not always carry over to easy decoding of words, pull-out isolated drill of morphology or vocabulary does not always result in effective and easy communication. LSA can explore and quantify the progress a student is making in application of language skills in the natural context of the skills.

It is important to monitor communication performance at reasonable intervals, but when frequently tested, students tend to simply "learn the test." Yet, it is necessary to use the same measure over time to document performance so that changes can be attributed to the student's development rather than to a new test procedure. LSA offers an opportunity to gather and analyze unlimited samples without fear of biasing the outcome. With frequent interactions, students relax with the examiner and provide samples of greater spontaneity and consistency. Examiners should vary the topics of discussion to keep the task interesting.

LSA provides a mechanism to monitor change over several years so that past data can be compared with current performance. The three-year M-team re-evaluation cycle is one example of the need for measures that can be performed consistently over many years and yield interpretable data.

Monitoring the progress of children who currently receive services allows SLPs to document changes in performance that may require alterations in the intervention program. When the child appears to meet the criteria for intervention goals, LSA can document generalization because of the opportunity for comparison of the results with the

Reference Database (RDB). These data may become part of a series of performance measures defining exit criteria.

LSA provides a powerful method to aid SLPs in monitoring changes in performance, supported by the RDB of typically developing children. The monitoring of children's progress is vital to focused intervention services. Speech and language services for children are costly, and require the implementation of methods that guide changes in intervention programs as well as procedures that ensure services are provided to only those children who truly require them. LSA will be useful in both of these efforts. Clinicians who consistently use LSA have found six different patterns of disordered expressive language performance. These patterns have, in turn, produced the focus for developing unique intervention strategies. The characterization and easy identification of these different types will be helpful in using LSA.

Recent Discoveries

In 1982, a group of Wisconsin SLPs from the Madison Metropolitan School District, who routinely use LSA, met to deliberate the question of whether or not language disorders were all alike or if there were distinct types. When indicating different types of expressive language disorders that were prevalent in their caseloads, SLPs discovered an amazing uniformity in their responses. They consistently distinguished six types of language disorders and also consistently described the specific performance differences in each. Only one is grounded in developmental delay. The other five are revealed in disordered language performance; that is, unorganized or confusing language production marked by various error patterns. Together, the six reflect a variety of productive language problems that are the product of perceptual and cognitive deficits, adaptations to everyday communication environments as well as responses to a variety of intervention programs. The focus on language production suggests that direct analysis of students' talking in various speaking conditions is critical for the development of appropriate intervention. Language comprehension deficits may or may not accompany each of the six disorder types. Each of the types of productive language deficits will be reviewed with a brief example transcript to provide a "feel" for the nature of these children.

Transcript Notation Key

C	=	Child utterance
E	=	Examiner utterance
()	=	mazes. All material in parenthesis are called (mazes), for example, false starts, repetitions and reformations
*	=	omitted word or part word
/	=	used to mark bound morphemes and contractions, for example, jump/ed (regular past)
:03etc	=	pause time in seconds
>	=	abandon utterance
X	=	Unintelligible word or segment
3S	=	Third person singular
/Z	=	possessive

1.   Utterance Formulation Problems

This narrative sample is from a boy, 8.5 years of age, who exhibits mazes that represent formulation problems. Utterance formulation is distinctly characterized by false starts, "(ah, th-) a girl"; repetitions, "(The boy, The boy) The boy went home"; or reformations, "(The boy is) The boys are riding their bikes." Many of the mazes in utterances could be interpreted as an inability to retrieve the appropriate word, though the majority are the result of utterance formulation problems. The length of his utterances is longer than the average eight year old, so he is capable of speaking for long periods of time. Yet he has difficulty completing the desired message. His mean length of utterance (MLU) is two standard deviations above the mean for children his age, which is typical of children with formulation problems. He is attempting to retell the story of "Rumpelstiltskin."

Mazes

Maze is a term which refers to a set of behaviors in speech that include
- false starts,
- repetitions, and
- reformations.

Mazes appear in the speech of children and adults when the oncoming spoken idea is undeveloped, uncertain, or complicated. Mazes may be as simple as "ums" or "ers" that do not interfere with or disrupt communication, unlike those presented in Figure 2. Everyone produces some mazes in their speech, but when produced frequently, mazes may directly indicate problems with utterance formulation or word finding.

■   Figure 2

C: (Um) he/'s the guy that make/3s (hi* um um the)>
C: He make/3s hay out of (gold) gold and (he he he) he uses/3s (um) something to spin it around with.
C: (And) because (um) the king (was was was wan*) want/ed to be greedier, so he said (um) "(do*) spin (th*) this wheel (and ma*) and make the hay out of gold."
E: Ok.
E: Why don't you tell me what happened first in the story.
C: (Um:04) well there was, something (like li*) like he was (um:03)>
C: (Well he, well he) well when he was/n't there, (um um) the lady was guess/ing his name, (and sh*) and he jump/ed up and down and say no no that was/n't, his name.
C: But at the end (he) she said (is her na*) is his name (rump*) Rumpelstiltskin?
C: (And) and (um, and then he he he ble*) then (um he he) he blew himself in half.

2.   Word Finding Problems

This child, who is 8.5 years of age, is telling the story of "Goldilocks and the Three Bears." Word finding problems are characterized by mazes that are *single word reformulations*, like "The boys (ran) rode to school"; or word choice errors, like, "The huge (cage) lifted the steel (barn) beam." Notice that his mazes are shorter and generally precede word choice changes. It appears that he frequently leaves out words as if he cannot retrieve them from memory. He also creates circumlocutions, which reflects an inability to provide sequence and order to a narrative. For example, this student returns to the element of eating in the story, even when that part of the narrative is no longer relevant.

Figure 3

E: Then what happen/ed?
: :02
C: (Um) :02 then they went up to the rocking chair/s and (ma* they) :03 father bear *said "somebody *has been (eat/ing) sit/ing in my chair."
E: Mhm.
C: And mamabear said "somebody *has been (eat/ing in my chair and by a) sit/ing by my chair.
C: And (um) babybear *said "somebody *has been eat/ing">
C: No.
C: "Sit/ing on my (p*) chair and someone broke it.
C: And so they went upstairs (and) :02 and grandpabear said "somebody *has been (si*) sit/ing in my bed."
C: And grandm*>
C: Nope.
; :03
C: Mamabear said "somebody *has been (see*) sleep/ing in my bed."
C: And (b*) little babybear (s*) *said "somebody *has been sleep/ing in my bed and there she is."
C: Then (when they) when (wi*) little>
; :02
C: With>
E: Are you try/ing to remember the girl/z name?
E: Goldilocks.
C: Goldilocks waked up and saw the threebears and she runned without her necklace.
C: And (sh*) her shoe.

3. Rate Problems

The conversational sample below is from a child 8.8 years of age with a rate of speech that is more than two standard deviations above the mean. There are two kinds of rate problems, characterized by either children who do not talk very much and take a great deal longer to produce a standard transcript of 100 utterances than their peers, or children who are oral "speed demons" but produce a sample without content. Children with both of these rate problems tax their listener's comprehension to the point where no one wants to talk with them. Other rate problems include long pauses between and within utterances. Children who use this "pause strategy" may be suffering from severe word finding or utterance formulation problems and prefer to pause rather than talk their way through classroom interaction. Unfortunately, teachers sometimes perceive these students as uncooperative. Frequent pauses are evident rather than mazes. The rate of speech cannot be clearly expressed in written form; the rate data from the reference database (Appendix A) provide the objective criteria for rate of speech for the first time. The content that the child attempts to express in the following sample is not clear, and the examiner finds it difficult to understand the student. The child is attempting to describe a science activity on eggs which the class had conducted for the past month. Accelerated rate, along with sparse or inappropriate message content, are the primary diagnostic indicators for placing this child in this category.

Figure 4

E: Where you doing an experiment?
C: Mhm
E: Tell me about it.
C: See when I crack/ed the egg open I had to take the yolk out out of the egg and put it in the bowl.
C: And we did/n't make an egg, but I could/v'e made a egg out of *it if I has a fork and a stove and a pot.
E: Then what did you do?
C: Then we had this little tube and at the end it was real big.
C: It had a cannon thing in it.
E: It had a what thing?
C: It was a big old machine we had.
C: We had to get some little piece/s that we made and we stuck it on there.
C: (Then) then we would pour egg in it.
C: Then it/'s sposta blow up and it did.
E: It did?
C: Yeah but not fire and smoke.
C: It just said pow.
C: But everybody had to stay away from it because i/'m the only one who knew what I was do/ing.
E: Excuse me, what blew up?

4. Pragmatic or Discourse Problems

The example transcript below is from a 5.4 year old child who is discussing dogs with the examiner. Note the frequent topic shifts, and the failure to regulate new and old information. This category contains a range of problems in the social use of language. Some problems arise in the relationship between utterances: topic maintenance, turn taking, and

10

the relation of new to old information during conversation. Problems exist in other speaking contexts as well: narration, object description, relation of events (storytelling), and logical argument. Behaviors associated with social appropriateness, which are usually attributed to social affective or personality disorders, are also in this category.

Figure 5

C: They got ear/s and soft.
C: Their headache.
C: And they got a tail
C: (My) I got two dog/s and one/z name is (um) shepherd and the name is Casey.
C: They/'re friend/s.
C: I like friend/s because some day/s dog/s are talky, barky or>
C: I don/'t wanna to (ah) just make the word/s are>
C: To make dog/s are>
C: Their bones are in their>
C: They could talk out to you.
C: Are you one that talk/3s?
C: The dog.
C: And he say/3s dog or something.
C: Someday (dog) dog trip/s are (t*) like hunter/s or shepherd/s or rabit/s.

5. Semantic or Reference Deficits

The transcript below is from a girl 4.9 years of age, retelling the story of "Little Red Riding Hood." What follows is a confused series of utterances that have little to do with the story even though she is both familiar with the story and looking at the picture book while retelling the tale. Hypothetically, limited vocabulary and an inability to make specific reference are her basic problems. These reference deficits focus on the word and utterance level, where semantic deficits at the word level are revealed by small vocabularies or the frequent use of universal pronouns and other words of indefinite reference like "things," "stuff," and "all that." At the utterance level, message content is confused and unclear. The examiner must determine whether the problems are based on inaccurate knowledge; or whether the confusing or often non-existent relationship among ideas expressed in sentences are the result of deficits in syntax or semantics; or whether the problems are the result of lexical deficits that produce unique adaptations of word use.

Figure 6

```
E:  (Le*) Tell me about the story of Little Red Riding Hood.
:    :03
C:  (Um) mommy good but>
;    :07
C:  (But) :03 daddy is but mommy and the kis/s>
C:  And mommy eat/ed [ew:ate] his lunch and that stuff.
C:  But>
C:  And that stuff.
;    :08
C:  Mommy and daddy and that stuff.
C:  And kid/s and mommy and that stuff.
C:  (And) and that stuff.
C:  But>
;    :05
C:  Well mommy fly but the bird fly/ed and it happen.
C:  And mommy start/3s to read it and stuff.
;    :02
C:  But the man x and mommy fly and gonna x.
C:  And then mommy fly/ed ain't gonna work x x.
C:  And mommy word/ed and mommy got it.
C:  (And dad) and SantaClaus could too.
;    :02
C:  Mommy have [ew:has] toy/s and SantaClaus *does too.
;    :04
C:  Xx SantaClaus said.
C:  SantaClaus said that.
C:  (And m*) and one and x.
C:  I wanna turn the page next.
C:  Me.
;    :04
C:  But that stuff>
```

6. Delayed Development

The performance data for these variables can be found in Appendix A. The child who produced the narrative transcript below is 7.10 years of age. Her performance is more than one standard deviation below the mean on all three developmental indicators. The relative low frequency of mazes and errors supports the categorization of developmental delay for this child.

Delayed development is characterized by language performance which falls significantly below the mean on variables that have documented high correlations with chronological age in children three to 13 years of age, such as mean length of utterance (MLU), Total Words, and the Number of Different Words. Mean length of utterance is the average length of utterances produced in a sample of 100 child utterances; Total Words is simply the total number of words produced in a sample of 100 utterances; and the Number of Different Words is the number of different words the child produces in 100 utterances.

This child had an MLU of 5.81 versus 7.17 for the average seven year old. She produced 515 total words in her language sample versus 648 for typically developing seven-year-old children, and she produced 152 different words versus an average of 190 for seven year olds.

■ Figure 7

E: Do you know the story of the Three Bears?
C: Mmm, yeah I have the book of that.
E: Ok, tell me that story.
C: (Um) there was a (puppy) papa and the mother and the baby.
E: Ok.
E: Then what.
C: Then they went in the woods.
E: They did?
E: Tell me some more.
C: And then the girl come/3s in the house and none was in there.
E: Mhm.
C: And the girl was knock/ing on the door.
E: Mhm.
C: And non/'s there.
C: And :03 she ate all the papa/z and mother/z and baby/z food.
E: She did?
E: What happened/ed next?
C: Then they come [ew:came] home.
C: They saw (um) the (s*) stuff.
C: Then she sat on the chair.
C: Mother/*z, papa/z.
C: And babybear/z chair broke.
E: Really?
E: Oh, and then what?
C: Then then she try/ed mama/z bed.
C: Papa/z bed.
C: (She pry*) she try/ed the kid/z one/s.
C: And she lik/3s (the kid/z) the kidbear/*z (um) bed.
E: Mhm.
C: And (they wo*) she wokedup and she went out the window.

Summary

These six types of language disorders belong to clinical categories of measurement and assessment. In more general terms, LSA can help children by its ability to
- substantiate the identification of Exceptional Educational Needs (EEN).
- describe productive language disorders to focus intervention efforts.
- document production disorders identified by teachers in children who perform well on standardized tests.

- document productive language proficiency in children who perform poorly on standardized measures of language performance.
- monitor effectiveness of language intervention in a variety of speaking conditions.
- potentially provide a culturally sensitive method for differentiating language difference from language disorder.

Although the field work has not yet culminated in strong documentation or cogent research, the categories are clinically valid by virtue of the fact that SLPs clearly recognize examples of these types of disorders on a regular basis. The measurement indicators are open to further refinement. The strength of LSA lies in its utility to describe any aspect of language performance that the SLP can define. The flexibility of LSA provides opportunity to use quantitative methods comparing individual performance with that of peers, and clinical judgment to interpret language performance and develop an intervention plan. The recognition of the complexity of the problem and the development of assessment tools that will allow description of developmental progress as well as deficits in performance encourages more consistent and appropriate placement.

References

Aram, D. M., B. L. Ekelman, and J. E. Nation. "Preschoolers with Language Disorders: Ten Years Later." *Journal of Speech and Hearing Research* 27 (1984), pp. 232-244.

Miller, J. "Assessing Children's Language Behavior: A Developmental Process Approach." In *The Basis of Language Intervention*. Ed. R. L. Schiefelbusch. Baltimore, MD: University Park Press, 1978, pp. 228-268.

Miller, J. F. *Assessing Language Production in Children: Experimental Procedures.* Austin, TX: PRO-ED, 1981.

Schery, T. K. "Correlates of Language Development in Language Disordered Children." *Journal of Speech and Hearing Disorders* 50 (1985), pp. 73-83.

Weiner, P. "The Value of Follow-up Studies." *Topics in Language Disorders* 5.3 (June 1985), pp. 78-92.

Language Sampling

Introduction

Collecting a language sample is the first crucial step in the LSA process. The object is to obtain a representative sample of the child's spontaneous language. The term "representative" refers to both reliability (the degree to which repeated samples are similar in content) and validity (the degree to which the sample represents the child's productive language ability). Only if SLPs record a representative sample will they be able to reliably interpret the child's performance as an index of linguistic knowledge. Current research in Wisconsin and clinical experience indicates that LSA is the only truly valid index of productive language performance. (Miller, 1991)

This chapter will focus on three parts of the LSA process:
- getting children to talk with spontaneity,
- creating representative samples, and
- recording samples for later transcription.

Each of these topics will provide specific methods to improve LSA skills, increase the reliability of samples collected, and ensure the validity of results.

Encouraging Spontaneous Interaction

Children will talk about everything. They make comments, requests, or demands about things they want or ideas that interest them. Children also respond to requests or demands that adults or other children make of them. The basic goal of talking is communication: sharing ideas by exchanging messages. Children understand this part of the talking game early in their development. Children are more likely to converse if they believe others are really interested in what they have to say. If they doubt a listener's sincerity, younger children may simply refuse to play the "talking game"; older children may cooperate but provide only minimal responses that do not reflect their communicative ability. The child who has difficulties is usually quite reticent and requires an environment of trust to achieve optimal communication. How can the SLP create this environment and gather the most representative sample of a student's productive language skills?

Collecting a Representative Sample

Interaction, the relationship established between the adult and the child, is basic to language sample collection. SLPs must relinquish their authoritative role and offer themselves instead as communication partners to the child.

Miller (1981) notes that the first few minutes of the language sample interaction are critical because they establish the integrity of the communicative interaction for the session. If the session begins well, the subsequent interaction will progress smoothly and fluently and should be fun. If the SLP fails to establish a comfortable rapport with the child, the resulting language sample will be strained and will lack the necessary spontaneity to function as a valid index of the child's productive language performance. Sometimes, it helps to inform the child of the purpose of the session, demonstrating how the tape recorder works and suggesting that the child listen to the tape when the sample collection is finished. Interest in the recording equipment will quickly fade as the child focuses on the conversation.

Miller (1981) suggests four variations in style that can be used, depending upon the status and age of the child to be recorded, to begin a recording session. These styles quickly establish shared interests for children who have difficulty interacting with adults.

- **Say nothing** beyond the initial friendly greetings for the first five minutes. This approach is particularly effective for children who are recalcitrant or self-conscious about their speech.
- **Parallel play** with little talking during the first few minutes. Any talking done by the examiner is directed at the toys rather than at the child. This approach has been effective with young children functioning at 30 months or below on cognitive tasks.
- **Interactive play** with little talking during the first few minutes. Toys can be shared by simply announcing, "I'm going to play with my gas station, you can play with it too." This approach is effective with children of cognitive level of three to five years.
- **Interactive play without introduction.** The SLP and child work together drawing pictures or molding play dough. Participation and discussion can be invited after the activity is underway. (This has been successfully used for children between three and nine years of age.)

Note that these activities generally reflect developmental characteristics and will have to be modified to meet the child's perceptual and motor abilities.

Miller (1981) lists the following suggestions in establishing and maintaining a productive communicative interaction:
- **Be enthusiastic:** Use smiles, vocal inflection, and eye contact.
— Generate a friendly demeanor.
- **Be patient:** Allow the child space and time to perform.
— Do not be afraid of pauses.
— Do not overpower the child with requests or directions.
- **Listen and follow the child's lead:** Help maintain the child's focus (topic and meaning) with immediate responses, comments, and questions.
— Use open-ended prompts and questions when possible: tell me more, then what happened?
— Add new information where appropriate.
— Maintain the child's pace, do not rush on to the next topic or direction.
- **Value the child:** Recognize the child's comments as important and worth undivided attention.
— Do not patronize the child.
— Demonstrate unconditional positive regard by nodding to show agreement and interest, and maintaining eye contact.
- **Do not play the fool:** Pay attention as if it were an adult conversation.
— Show interest with eye contact, facial expression, and vocal inflection.
— Refrain from asking questions with obvious answers.
- **Learn to think like a child:** Remember that children's perspectives vary, depending upon levels of cognitive development.
— Be alert to a child's awareness of action, time, space, and cause, and recognize how that knowledge affects the sample.
— Adapt language to the level of the child's development of language.
— Shorten utterances (if needed), simplify vocabulary, and reduce complexity.

It is important to remember that these suggestions are relevant for all children regardless of their cultural, economic, or language background, or their cognitive, physical, or speech and language differences. The goal is to provide children a maximum opportunity to communicate to the best of their ability. It is the SLP's responsibility to evaluate what the child can do communicatively under various speaking conditions. This task requires clinical judgment and knowledge of the language complexity that children understand and use at various ages. In this sense, there is no substitute for experience in talking with children of various ages and ability levels. But even the most experienced SLP must guard against any possible behavior that would inhibit the child's performance.

Conversational Versus Narrative Samples

Oral communication serves a variety of purposes: to exchange information in conversation; to share stories; to retell familiar stories or legends; to share TV programs or movies; to sell something; to express needs; to persuade, comment, or question. These different purposes are referred to as speaking contexts. Miller's research has documented that children of the same age apply their language differently relative to the speaking context. Research and clinical practice focus on two speaking conditions, conversation and narration. SLPs in Wisconsin have collected considerable data on children's performance in the speaking contexts of conversation and narration; data which will be reviewed here as well as in the interpretive sections of this guide. Children can successfully engage in conversations long before they can be expected to produce a reasonable narrative. Narratives cannot be expected before children reach three years of age and even then would be quite primitive with only a few utterances per episode. Establishing two well-defined speaking contexts, conversation and narration, for initial assessments will allow the comparison of an individual child's performance to those of other children the same age, as well as follow the individual child's progress over time.

It will be important to examine the child's performance within a range of speaking conditions in order to explore the breadth and depth of the child's productive language ability. Figure 8 graphically illustrates increasingly complex speaking contexts expected of a child at various age or developmental levels. It begins with conversation and proceeds to several types of narrative or storytelling. Conversation, as the first speaking context, is located at the top of the matrix in Figure 8 because at the very beginning of learning language, children can be engaged in conversations. During free play between parent and child these conversations give beginning language learners the opportunity to produce spontaneous language. Children up to about age three are most comfortable with their parents, and parents know what their children like to talk about and what experiences they like to share. The language produced in this context generally focuses on the here and now, on the children's toys and on the activities in which they are currently engaged. As children get older, they can use language to transcend time and space. Therefore, SLPs who interact with children three years of age or older should introduce topics that are absent in time and space giving the child the opportunity to reveal and express the space, time, and causal relationships that they understand in their language. Samples collected in this way are more diverse because the range of topics can be varied. This will increase the likelihood that children will use complex sentences and vocabulary in their utterances to talk about objects, actions, and relations.

Figure 8 presents narration as the second speaking context. Narratives, the telling or retelling of stories, events, or experiences, play a substantial role in the educational process: learning to read and displaying acquired information relies heavily on narrative abilities. The matrix in Figure 8 contains a number of narrative contexts, the most com-

Figure 8 ■

Language Sample Contexts by Age or Developmental Level

Ages

| | 1 | 2 | 3 | 4 | 5 | 6 | 7 | 8 | 9 | 10 | 11 | 12 | 13 | 14 | 15 | 16 | 17 | 18 |

Speaking Contexts

Conversation
- Parent-child or pathologist-child interaction in play setting.
- Introduce topics absent in time and space at three years of age. Focus topics on time and cause as age increases.

Narration
- Report an event, relate a personal experience. Relate a TV program episode, movie, or play.

Storytelling
- Retell familiar story, legend, or fable.
- Retell the "Bus Story" picture story task.*
- Invent own fictional stories.
- Retell stories from reading textbooks with graded content.

Description
- Describe picture.
- Describe functional use of objects.
- Describe how to play a favorite game.
- Compare and contrast objects or events.
- Describe daily activities, "what you do from the time you get up until you go to bed."

Academic Tasks
- Classroom interaction.
- Small groups; problem-solve, discuss specific academic areas: science, social studies, history.

Comparing oral and written language
- Storytelling. Description tasks.
- Academic tasks.

* For a description of the "Bus Story," see Bishop, D. and A. Edmundson, "Language-Impaired 4 year olds: Distinguishing Transient from Persistent Impairment." *Journal of Speech and Hearing Disorders* 52 (1987), p. 156-173.

mon for school-age children being the retelling of a favorite story or television program. This context provides the child with maximum opportunity to retell a story successfully because such stories require a beginning, a middle, and an ending, all of which move through the appropriate chronology.

As language performance expectations advance, the SLP can introduce various speaking contexts designed to tax the child's language performance to the maximum. Such activities may include instructing the child to explain the rules of a favorite game. This task is quite difficult because it generally requires the child to produce a set of rules that are applied under specific conditions. The child must also accurately relate the chronology of the game sequence. The use of relative and temporal language is complex, and language-impaired children frequently have difficulty with such tasks. Older language-impaired children may have difficulty with written language that parallels their oral language problems. For example, a child who says, "He goed," may also write "He goed." The same strategies used in language sample analysis have been used successfully to analyze written language.

Collecting Samples for Comparison with the RDB

In establishing criterion reference data for school-age children, *conversation* and *narration* offer SLPs the broadest opportunity to analyze productive language skills that are relevant to educational settings. Both sampling conditions offer the opportunity to analyze vocabulary, syntax, and semantics, as well as the unique features of each: taking turns; maintaining topic; responding to contingent speech in conversation; maintaining story structure; ordering of events; and relating story characters (for narration). As mentioned previously Miller, the Madison Metropolitan School District, and CESA 9, in cooperation with the Wisconsin Department of Public Instruction, developed a database in Wisconsin (see Appendix A) over the past eight years for children between three and 13 years of age. To replicate sampling conditions that were used in establishing the database, the specific directions used with the children can be found in Figure 9.

 Figure 9

Language Sampling Protocol for Collecting Conversation and Narrative Samples

Conversation: 15 minutes in length.
Elicit language related to ongoing events during the following activities:
1) Playing with clay
2) Activities from classroom units

Introduce at least one topic absent in time and space from the sampling condition.
1) Holidays, what did you do, will you do
2) Family activities, visits, locations, etc.
3) Family pets
4) How to play a favorite game.

Questions and prompts to facilitate talk in conversational contexts:
The following questions and prompts have been used effectively in the past. Do not limit yourself to these examples, use what ever works for you.

Conversation: Clay
"I've bought some clay for us to play with today."
"I wonder what we could make together?"
Follow the child's suggestions, request directions, etc. or
"I'm going to make ___. What do I need to do it?" or comment on the child's activity with the clay.

Conversation: Classroom activities, etc.
"Tell me about some of the things you've been doing in school lately." Ask about specific classroom units. "Did you do anything special for Halloween (etc.)?" Tell me about that. "Are you going to do anything special for Christmas?"
"Are you going to visit your grandma, grandpa?" "Where do they live?" "How do you get there" "What do you do there?"
"Do you have any pets at home?" "Tell me about them" "What do you have to do to take care of them?"

Narration: 15 minutes in length.
1) Tell a favorite story
2) Retell an episode from a TV program.
3) Retelling a familiar story, "Goldilocks and the Three Bears," "Little Red Riding Hood," the "Three Little Pigs." Picture prompts may be used only after every attempt has been made to elicit spontaneous speech.

Questions and prompts to facilitate talk in narrative contexts:
Narration TV
"Do you watch TV?"
"What programs do you like?"
"Tell me about that one, I haven't seen it"
"What happened on the last one you watched?"
"Do you ever watch (insert current programs likely to be of interest)?"

Narration story
"Do you know any stories?"
"What is one of your favorite stories?"
"Oh, I don't know that one very well, will you tell it?"
"Do you know Little Red Riding Hood, etc.?" "Ooo, tell me about that one."
Use prompts as necessary, but make them open ended . . . . "Can you tell me more?" "What else happened?"
You can use picture books for the familiar stories for the three year olds, if necessary. Have books for the stories you think the children will know.

Transcription Aids

Write down any unusual names that are spoken during the session. Names can be difficult to transcribe because they are unfamiliar. Keep glossing to a minimum in order to maintain the flow of conversation. Any gains made in intelligibility may be offset by loss of conversation or narrative flow. Please make notes of any unusual events that may transpire during the recording session, interruptions, tape recorders stopping or failing. It will be useful to keep a log book for this purpose. Record each child's name on a page and summarize, after the session, comments about performance or weird happenings that may play a role in interpreting the session.

Instructions for Figure 9 require SLPs to use the basic principles outlined in the interaction portion of this section. The narrative context is difficult for children three years of age or younger, and they need continual prompts from the SLP, in the form of new stories, to gain as much language as possible.

Transcript Length

Samples should contain 100 complete and intelligible utterances. Tape-recording 15 minutes of conversation or narration will usually ensure a sufficient number of utterances or a usable transcript of 12 minutes. It is important to note that children with language production difficulties will take longer to produce 100 utterances than children without difficulties. Children nine years of age or older usually will produce 100 utterances in approximately three to four minutes. Thus the amount of talking per unit of time is of diagnostic significance and explains why the amount of time elapsed for the sample is recorded. The length of sample is concerned with two variables; the number of utterances that the child produces and the elapsed time of the sample. The Reference Database in Appendix A provides 100 complete and intelligible utterance characterizations of child performance at each age level, as well as a 12-minute characterization of performance for temporal variables.

The use of 100 complete and intelligible utterances is somewhat arbitrary. Some language analysis formats require 25, 30, or 50 utterances. One hundred utterances allows the child to display a variety of language abilities. Other researchers have investigated the numbers of utterances that are required for "stable" analysis. For example, Bruce Tomblin and his colleagues at the University of Iowa note that 250 utterances are required before they can perform a stable Developmental Sentence Scoring analysis. (Lee, 1974) The language produced in the samples can vary depending on the following: the instructions given to the child; the examiner's skill in introducing the same kinds of topics; and the context in which the child is to respond. The degree to which a sampling context is established and controlled will determine the degree to which a language sample is a reliable and valid index of what the child knows. One hundred utterances is not going to tell SLPs everything about the child's productive language; however, it is a sufficient number to be of diagnostic significance for basing decisions about exceptional educational needs.

Do not assume that the sample is always 100 percent reliable and valid. People are fallible and capable of collecting data that is not reliable nor a valid index of the child's performance. An SLP must consider variables that effect a child's performance: hearing; vision; cognition; and experiential background. It is also important to keep in mind that LSA data should be interpreted within the context of other collected assessment data.

Figure 10

Equipment and Recording Considerations Checklist

The purpose of this section is to review the requirements for creating the highest quality recording possible. The following list will remind the SLP of factors to consider before recording a session.

Tape Recorder
- ❏ select a high quality recorder
- ❏ consider an external jack
- ❏ estimate the need for service and repair
- ❏ consider portability
- ❏ judge the recorder's durability

Microphones
- ❏ use an external microphone

Tape Selection
- ❏ high quality
- ❏ durability (for repeated playing)
- ❏ maximum of 60 minutes
- ❏ minimum of 30 minutes

Reduce Interference by Considering:
- ❏ ambient noise
- ❏ room's acoustic quality
- ❏ distance between microphone and speaker
- ❏ direction of the microphone
- ❏ surface (table top)
- ❏ loudness of the child's voice
- ❏ non-speech noises the child makes (clicking pencil, drumming fingers)

Check Equipment before Meeting with Child
- ❏ be familiar with the recorder
- ❏ be familiar with other types of recorders and microphones if alternate equipment is necessary
- ❏ record the child's name
- ❏ record date
- ❏ record the school's name
- ❏ play back
- ❏ test for level and clarity

Written Documentation to be Provided with Tape
- ❏ child's name
- ❏ date of testing
- ❏ sampling condition
- ❏ date of birth
- ❏ school
- ❏ use code names for confidentiality (when needed)

23

Summary

The sampling phase of LSA determines the language content that will be available for analysis. The sampling process requires considerable clinical skill and sensitivity in order to obtain a valid and reliable sample. While defining the speaking context and indicating ways to optimize the child's verbal production will help reduce variability, sampling remains an artistic enterprise. The SLP uses every means available to encourage the child to perform. The more the child exhibits difficulty, the more clinical skill will be required to get the child to demonstrate individual language and communication ability.

References

Lee, L. *Developmental Sentence Analysis.* Evanston, IL: Northwestern University Press, 1974.

Miller, J. "Quantifying Productive Language Disorder." In *Research on Child Language Disorders: A Decade of Progress.* Ed. J. Miller. Austin, TX: PRO-ED, 1991, pp. 211-220.

Miller, J. F. *Assessing Language Production in Children: Experimental Procedures.* Austin, TX: PRO-ED, 1981.

3

Transcription

Introduction

Transcription is the process used:
- to preserve a child's speech in written form.
- to code a child's speech so that SLPs can analyze it in a variety of ways.
- to make the speech readable, and thus easily *accessible* to anyone interested in the child's language production, including parents.

Traditionally, the speech and language pathologist assumed sole responsibility for the entire process of gathering information: the interaction and the recording, the transcription of recorded speech to paper, and the analysis of the language sample. Currently, Wisconsin is developing transcription labs in some areas where specially trained clerical personnel transcribe the recorded language samples. This effort enables SLPs to increase the amount of time they have to interact with the child and to analyze the language sample, and decrease the time-consuming responsibility of transcription.

Literally thousands of decisions are made at the sound, word, and utterance level during the transcription of every language sample. The goal is to represent exactly what the *child says* with as little transcriber modification as possible. As competent speakers of English, listeners tend to correct errors and miscues, and inadvertently regularize the child's language. Transcribers must inhibit this tendency and work toward recognizing cues from the language that will reveal the child's intentional utterances and word meanings.

Utterances, for example, are cued by a child's use of intonation and pause. Decisions about word meanings require a combination of cues: an accurate recording of the sound pattern produced; an interpretation based on the transcriber's knowledge of both English and the topic of conversation and shared knowledge of the world between the transcriber and the child. Dimensions like speech intelligibility are greatly influenced by familiarity with the speaker, therefore the transcriber should review earlier coding after gaining greater familiarity with the child. The success of the transcription process, and the resulting analysis and interpretation, depends on the skill of the transcriber to create a faithful rendition of the recorded sample.

A standard transcription format, with flexible rules for various options, as well as training and experience will give the transcription process an accuracy of 95 percent or higher across SLPs in the state of Wisconsin. The remainder of this chapter introduces the standard format, transcription conventions for a wide range of linguistic and non-linguistic behaviors, and the models of the transcription process.

The Basic Goals of the Format

Creating a transcript of a language sample involves a great deal of time and effort. The transcription format should meet several conditions in order to take advantage of this effort. The overriding goal is to establish one standard format that can be used, read, and understood by public school SLPs for current analysis and others which may be desired in the future. In meeting this goal, the authors of this guide considered several other goals extremely important in optimizing the use of LSA. First, the transcript should be readable: *anyone*—parents, teachers, and administrators—should be able to read the transcript and understand what transpired during the recording session. Meeting this goal allows SLPs the additional benefit of sharing LSA data with parents and school personnel.

Another goal is to create a flexible format that provides conventions for recording all possible verbal and accompanying non-verbal behaviors in the event that multilevel analyses are needed. The use of all transcription conventions is optional, providing the flexibility to transcribe only what is necessary for analysis. One of the most flexible transcription features is a convention for coding words or utterances using square brackets, which appears like the following: [code]. This feature can be used for coding anything about individual words or utterances, like the range of meanings expressed by propositions or communicative intentions of utterances, or errors at the word or utterance level.

This mechanism offers the transcriber the opportunity, to not only document the child's developmental progress, but to evaluate error patterns that are characteristic of a variety of language deficits. The more detail that is included in the transcript of the language sample, the greater the variety and specificity of the analyses which can be performed. If utterances of the conversational partner are included, for example, discourse or pragmatic analysis and responses to questions or other contingent speech can be analyzed. It is helpful and time efficient to know the required levels of analysis at the time of transcription.

The transcription format proposed in this guide is the same one used to create the Reference Database which uses the computer program, Systematic Analysis of Language Transcripts (SALT). The transcription conventions are appropriate and useful for doing analyses by hand since this transcription format does not require computer software for analysis. While SALT can be used to analyze transcripts in this format, other language analysis software programs have transcript convention conversion programs to reformat a SALT transcript to suit the program requirements. With the transcript format proposed here, transcription need only be done once whether analyses are to be done by hand or using a variety of computer programs. The method of analysis may depend on the specificity and depth of analysis desired.

Identifying Utterances and Words

During transcription, the initial identification of words and correct utterance segmentation is critical because identification is the fundamental component for all other analyses. Deciding what constitutes words and utterances for children with language impairments is not always a straightforward task because intelligibility and prosody may be impaired. These decisions, therefore, present the greatest challenge to the transcriber. Utterance segmentation is relatively easy as long as the child is producing only one utterance per speaking turn, that is child utterances precede and follow adult utterances, one by one. For example:

E So, what have you been doing in your classroom today?
C Play/ing with blocks.
E Play/ing with blocks?
C Big ones you can stand on.

Two utterance segmentation rules were used in the development of the reference database. The first rule uses intonation to define what constitutes an utterance. A falling intonation contour defines comments and statements. A rising intonation contour defines questions. The second rule uses pausing to identify utterances. A pause may or may not accompany a rising or falling intonation. Speakers, sensitive to pauses of greater than two seconds, generally interpret them as signals for turn changes. The consistent use of these segmentation rules is important for analysis. The calculation of mean length of utterance (MLU) depends directly on how utterances are segmented. In the transcript fragment above, the child produced two utterances. The first is three words and the second is six words, so the average or mean number of words in the two utterances is 9/2 = MLU of 4.5. If the child had not used a falling intonation contour after saying "Playing with blocks," or used a pause of greater than two seconds, then the second utterance, "big ones you can stand on," would have been added to the first to create a single nine word utterance. Obviously, the resulting MLU would be different. Mean length of utterance is an index of grammatical complexity. In general, as utterances get longer, they also get more complex.

The pause and intonation rules work consistently for identifying utterances through the phase of simple sentence development. Difficulties arise, however, when children conjoin utterances and produce complex sentences. Under these circumstances, segmentation of utterances occurs after the child produces one conjunction. For example, "We went to Grandma's house and my brother went too," would be considered a single utterance. But if the child adds, "We went to Grandma's house and my brother and my cousin went also," the final conjoined clause, "my cousin went also," would be considered a separate utterance. The intent of this rule is to avoid overly long utterances as a result of using multiple conjunctions like, "and then . . . and then . . . and then . . . ." This rule somewhat parallels Loban's (1976) grammatically-based rule for segmenting communication units. This guide's proposed format attempts to be sensitive to what the child intends even though grammatical knowledge may be limited or deficient.

Decisions about what constitutes a word are particularly critical for analyzing young children's, language production (until about age two). It is also relevant for analyzing the language of children who are cognitively disabled and functioning at the early stages of language development. The primary consideration for what constitutes a word is the child's consistent use, and the transcriber's consistent interpretation of that word. A "word" is in the ear of the listener. If a parent or person familiar with the child considers a production a word and assigns meaning to it, it functions as a word. The appropriate place to look for meaning is in the child's immediate environment. Children talk about what they experience and with whom they interact. Those familiar people and consistent events generally accompany consistent language input. These consistent people, events, and objects (associated with these events) are represented early in the language-learning process. It is extremely unlikely, if not impossible, for young children to represent objects and events with which they have not participated or not experienced directly.

Transcribing language samples of children with potential language impairment requires the transcriber to make decisions about the accuracy of production. Although transcription usually entails the written recording of a child's words and utterances, it also encompasses a transcriber's judgment about the accuracy of those productions in order to aid the analysis. For example, the child who says, "goed" instead of "went," may do so consistently. It is an important and informative aspect of the child's language production and therefore it must be coded in some way. The same is true for utterances that fail to convey the proper meaning or use erroneous grammatical structure (failure to maintain word order, use of the wrong word selection, or response to questions with the use of appropriate grammatical form but inappropriate content). These kinds of behaviors can go undetected if not marked at the time of transcription. Therefore, a limited set of codes should be inserted at the time of transcription. This will help the SLP analyze the language sample appropriately. These codes note that the child produced an error but do not require the transcriber to take the time to figure out the nature of the error. Those decisions are left to the SLP during the analysis process. Coding errors at the word and utterance level allows a variety of language errors to be identified so they will not be overlooked. This can be done with the following codes: word error [EW], utterance error [EU], and content (unclear) error [CU]. Error codes serve to expand the SLP's analytical options beyond the standard variables that note developmental progress. The SLP can also analyze utterances with errors to identify inappropriate use of language production.

Mazes

A second major coding-error category is mazes. It may not be appropriate to call mazes errors, but they are a major source of information about children's word and utterance formulation problems. A maze refers to any false start, repetition, or reformulation. When maze words are removed from the utterance, the remaining words can stand alone. It is important to code mazes so that they are not counted as part of the utterance; this excludes them from mean length of utterance counts and other similar analyses. At the same time, the mazes can be independently analyzed. Mazes are extremely important variables that identify formulation problems on the part of the speaker. For example, in Figure 11, line two reads, "He make/3s hay out of (gold) gold and (he he he) he use/es (um) something to spin it around with." The child produces three mazes, each marked by parentheses. The first is a repetition of "gold," the second a repetition of "he," and the last a filled pause, "um." Mazes also include false starts, "(the, the) a girl," and reformulations, "he (goed) went." The reference database documents these behaviors as frequent in normal subjects as well as in children with production language problems. Mazes become important diagnostically with increased frequency (more than 20 to 25 percent), increased number of words included in the maze (more than three to four), the position of the mazes (multiple versus one, and placement prior to the verb phrase or elsewhere in the utterance), and the number of mazes per utterance. The coding of mazes provides an opportunity to document problems associated with utterance formulation and word finding that would otherwise go undetected.

Standard Transcription Format

The transcription format is comprised of the standard conventions to record, in writing, the language sample. This improves SLP's ability to communicate with each other about specific children and to document children's progress over time in a consistent manner. Transcribing both the child's and the speaking partner's utterances provides opportunity to analyze language at the morpheme, word, utterance, and discourse levels. A detailed account of the SALT transcription conventions can be found in Appendix B. Please refer to this appendix if there is difficulty understanding any transcript conventions in the example transcripts in this guide. It is instructive to read through these conventions to appreciate how few of them are needed, and how readable the transcript is, even when a difficult language production problem exists. Figure 11 provides a brief example transcript.

Figure 11

Example Transcript

Child: Erin M.
Examiner: Kathy L.
Sex: Female
DOB: 5-9-77
DOE: 10-23-85
CA: 8;5
Context: Narration
School: Blue Valley Public Schools
+ [EU] = Error at the Utterance Level
+ [EW] = Error at the Word Level
+ [CU] = Content Unclear
= C   Retelling Rumpelstiltskin story.
-   0:00
C (Um) he/'s the guy that make/3s (hi* um um the)>
C He make/3s hay out of (gold) gold and (he he he) he use/3s (um) something to spin it around with.
C (And) because (um) the king (was was was wan*) want/ed to be greedier[EW], so he said (um) "(do) spin (th*) this wheel (and ma*) and make the hay out of gold."
E Ok.
E Why don't you tell me what happened first in the story.
C (Um :04) well there was, something (like li*) like he was (um :03)>
C (Well he, well he) well when he was/n't there, (um um) the lady was guess/ing his name, (and sh*) and he jump/ed up and down and say[e:said] no no that was/n't, his name.
C But at the end (he) she said (is her na*) is his name (Rump*) Rumpelstiltskin?
C (And) and (um, and then he he he ble*) then (um he he) he blew himself in half.
E Ok.
E Let's start this way chance.
E Once upon a time, there was>
C <(Um)>^
E <Can> you finish that sentence?
C (Um) I don't know.
E Once upon a time there was a>
C Man call/ed Rumpelstiltskin.
E Mhm.
C (And) and he want/ed (to have um) to make gold (for) for that woman (that) that she was go/ing to make [EU].
C (And) and she make[ew:made] all her promise/s [EU].
C (And then) and then she could keep the baby, (when when she, when it was a*) when she (ha*) had it at the end.
E Mhm.
E How did the story end?
C (Um um as ha*) as happy as she live/ed.
= C   Means to say "she live/ed happily ever after"?

E   Ok.
E   Who were the people in the story?
C   (Um) Rumpelstiltskin, a queen, a prince (and and the x) and the princess.
E   Tell me about the queen.
C   (Um) the queen (wa* want/ed to make) had to make the gold, so the king told her.
E   Tell me about the princess.
C   (Um) the princess (um um lo*) lock/ed her inside all alone when the strange man appear/ed (to) to make all the gold.
E   And tell me about the prince.
C   (Um he) he had (um to) to visit (th*) the king (and) and tell him all about the gold.
E   And tell me about Rumpelstiltskin.
C   (He he was a stra*) he was a strange man.
E   Why was he strange?
C   Because, he was like, (um i) with a hat and he had a beard.
C   And a mustache.
E   What did you like best about the story?
C   (Um) I like/ed that (um)>
C   It was very nice.
E   Can you tell me more?
C   (Um) and (there) well there could be a little bit of (:02 he* :02)>
C   Well, if I can think of it.
;   :04
C   I know, it/'s now (um) that (he) he become/3s strange at the end.
C   (Um and) and how it (end) end/ed (when when th*) when the prince told the king about (th*)the gold and lock/ed the princess in the room.
Total time elapsed: 4:27

The first two lines present the speakers' names and the letters that will be used thereafter to refer to who is talking. Figure 11 also provides information regarding the child's gender; date of birth, date of evaluation; chronological age; name of the school the child attends; and or any other information the SLP thinks is relevant. A consistent set of information helps the SLP when using the transcript in subsequent months and years. There is a starting time marker at the beginning of the transcript. At the end of the transcript, a similar time marker is inserted noting the total elapsed time of the transcript.

Computer programs, like SALT, will calculate automatically the number of words and utterances per minute, produced by the child, if the total elapsed time is given for the transcript. The transcript begins after the starting time marker. When using SALT "Cs" precede the child's utterances and "Es" are used to indicate the examiner's utterances. (See Appendix B.) The examiner's utterances are indented so that it is easier to read the child's utterances. If writing the transcript by hand, one may wish to use this notation system to improve readability of the transcript.

Transcription Time

Transcription time is generally a result of sample length, intelligibility, and the intactness of the child's language. A 15-minute language sample will take from an hour and fifteen minutes to two hours to transcribe depending upon the intelligibility of the child and the nature of the child's language disorder. As intelligibility decreases and/or the language impairment becomes more severe, transcription time increases. It is also important to remember that as children get older, they produce more language per unit of time. So a 12-year-old child can be expected to produce twice as much speech in 15 minutes as a five year old. While language-impaired children typically do not talk as much as children with normal language, one should expect to spend more time transcribing older children's samples compared to younger children.

Transcription Aids

Tape recorders can be used for recording and transcription. They require constant stopping, starting, and moving back and forth, in order to make sure that everything the child produces is transcribed. This very tedious process wears out tape recorders quickly. Consequently, over the last seven to eight years, speech and language programs have invested in machines that were originally used by secretaries for the transcription of letters and correspondence. These machines operate with standard cassettes and use foot pedals to free both hands for keyboard or handwritten entries. The foot pedal can be set so that when the tape is stopped, it automatically rewinds a specified number of words. This is a tremendous aid to transcription saving an estimated 30 to 40 percent of transcription time, and extending the life of tape recorders. See Appendix F for more information on cost effectiveness.

Models of the Transcription Process

The transcription process has traditionally been thought of as a negative part of the SLP's task in LSA. After recording the child's language in a particular context, the SLP requires a significant amount of time to transcribe and analyze the tape. An alternative model is a transcription laboratory. A transcription laboratory provides the transcription service for the SLP. The SLP tape records the sample and submits it to the laboratory. The laboratory transcribes it using standard conventions, and returns the transcript, including some basic analyses when computer analysis software is available. The SLP can then spend valuable time performing more detailed analyses and interpreting the results. This model allows the SLP to spend more time interpreting the data and designing a focused intervention sequence, and less on the routine and time-consuming task of transcription. SLPs have used this model for the last three years in the Madison Metropolitan School District, and the evaluation of its effectiveness has been outstanding. When the process began, the service was offered to all 52 SLPs in the Madison Metropolitan School District. By the end of the first year, 48 SLPs had used the lab and more than 520 tapes had been transcribed. The consistency of transcription improved communication within the district when children transferred between schools. It was also used to quantify progress within therapy. See Appendix F for more information on cost effectiveness.

Summary

In summary, transcription is the backbone of the language sample analysis. The consistency of the transcription format, the detail of the transcript, and the skill of the transcriber are all critical pieces to the final product of the language analysis itself.

References

Loban, W. O. *Language Development: Kindergarten Through Grade Twelve*. Urbana, IL: National Council of Teachers of English, 1976.

4

Analysis

Introduction

Analyzing a language sample is a time-intensive process, even with the aid of computers. A sample must be evaluated from various angles to distinguish the degree of delay or disordered performance, and then to evaluate selected levels of language performance (lexical, syntax, semantic, or pragmatic) for further evaluation. The SLP's goal is to spend time efficiently in order to effectively document productive language performance. This chapter on analysis will review a variety of general analyses relative to how they lead to the identification of major problem areas. Further detailed analyses of a transcript may be necessary to describe disorders in sufficient detail to develop an intervention plan. This efficient strategy will optimize the time required, so that SLPs perform only the necessary analyses. The measures included in this section cover a wide range of language performance areas, from indicators of developmental progress to the description of production errors, each capable of documenting specific areas of concern, and thus pointing to the direction of further analysis. In this section, discussion of the Reference Database (RDB) located in Appendix A is informational, not instructional. More specific instructions on how to read and use the RDB appear in the next section, "Interpretation."

Getting Started

Two methods are available for performing analysis from a transcript: pencil-and-paper or computer-assisted. Almost all of the analyses discussed in this section can be calculated by hand; some are just more complex and time-consuming to complete than others. Counting the number of different words can be done, but is tedious. Computers are better suited to these counting and sorting tasks, because they can perform them in seconds. The Reference Database in Appendix A interprets analysis performed by hand or by computer. The RDB requires only that the samples are taken under the same speaking conditions as the reference sample (see Section 2) and are of comparable length to the reference sample.

The following procedures have the power to document developmental progress as well as deficits in language structure and use. Methods for calculating each measure will accompany each description.

Measurements of Developmental Progress

LSA offers SLPs the opportunity to measure developmental progress. These measurements correlate to the student's age. There are three confirmed indicators of developmental progress for language performance that are derived from LSA data. These are: mean length of utterance (MLU) which is usually calculated in morphemes; the number of different words (NDW) produced in the transcript and calculated based on 100 complete and intelligible utterances; and the total number of words (TNW) produced in a transcript of a 12-minute duration. As the reader will recall, 12 minutes or 100 utterances is the length of each sample used in the Reference Database although SLPs are required to tape for 15 minutes to ensure a reliable sample. (Miller, 1990) These measures are indexes of developmental progress because each correlates highly with advances in chronological age. (Miller, 1991)

These three measures, MLU, NDW, TNW, all assess a different aspect of language performance. Each of these measures are a potential index of developmental progress in language production.

Mean Length of Utterance (MLU)

Mean length of utterance in morphemes is a general measure of syntactic development. Roger Brown and his students at Harvard University originally used it to define stage-like advances in syntactic development and argued that grammatical complexity must increase as utterance length increases. MLU also provides a convenient way of summarizing performance over a large number of utterances both within and between subjects.

Originally, professionals believed that MLU was useful only through the period of simple sentence development; that is, MLUs of four to five morphemes. The stability of MLU and its high correlation to age was demonstrated by Miller and Chapman (1991) for children with normal language and by Klee, et al (1989) for children with both normal language and disorders. Loban (1976) found mean length of utterance systematically increases through grades K-12. The Loban segmentation criteria provide a systematic, grammatically motivated set of rules that can be combined with Miller's (1981) segmentation rules. Together, these make possible the exploration of how MLU correlates to age in older children as well as how MLU relates to other general measures of language change.

Calculating Mean Length of Utterance

The following rules for calculating MLU are from Miller (1981) and are the same rules used to calculate MLU in the RDB.

• Prepare a transcript of child utterances as described in Section 3. The sample should follow the protocol for conversation or narration described in Figure 11, Section 3.

• Select the first 100 complete and intelligible utterances in the sample.

• Count the number of morphemes in each utterance.

• Find the total number of morphemes and divide by the number of utterances (400 morphemes by 100 utterances yield an MLU = 4.0).

Remember: A morpheme is the minimal meaningful unit of the language. Dog is a single morpheme, but dogs is two morphemes, **dog** plus **s**, noting more than one. The rules for determining morphemes follow Brown (1973). Consult Brown's text for answers to specific questions, but above all, be consistent within a transcript. The following are items that occur frequently and could affect MLU if not handled consistently:

• **Mazes** (false starts, repetitions, and reformulations) are to be marked and excluded from the MLU calculation. Refer to the maze calculation part of this section.

• **Compound words and multi-word titles** of books or movies are to be counted as one morpheme. If the child names a single thing, only one morpheme is credited regardless of how many morphemes are used to make the reference. Therefore, *The Three Bears* would be written as *TheThreeBears* and counted as only one morpheme.

• **All irregular past tense verbs** should be counted as single morphemes since evidence shows children relate these to the present form (went, saw, ran, did).

• **Diminutives** (doggie, mommy) and catenatives (gonna, wanna, hafta) are to be counted as one morpheme.

• **Auxiliaries** (is, have, will, can, must, and would) are to be counted as separate morphemes.

Number of Different Words (NDW) and Total Number of Words (TNW)

Miller (1991) has recently documented two additional measures as excellent indicators of developmental progress in language production. First, the number of different words (NDW) produced in a sample of standard length (100 complete and intelligible utterances in this guide's data) is a measure of general semantic progress or semantic diversity. Second, the total number of words (TNW) produced in a sample of standard length (12 minutes' transcript duration in this guide's data) is a more specific index of general language proficiency. The index of the total number of words reflects speaking rate, length of utterance, speech and motor maturation (Kent, 1976; 1984), utterance formulation ability, and word retrieval efficiency. One might expect the total number of words to vary from conversation to narration.

Calculating the Number of Different Words (NDW)

To calculate the number of different words, use the first 100 complete and intelligible child utterances in the transcript. Count all word roots as words, excluding words occurring in mazes. If one calculated MLU, count all morphemes that stand alone as word roots. Bound morphemes, -ed, -ing, -s, for example, are not counted. Each different word can be only counted once for this calculation regardless of how many different bound morphemes are used with it. **Go** and **went** are each counted; yet if **play**/ed and **play**/ing also appear, only **play** is counted.

Calculating the Total Number of Words (TNW)

Use the preceding rules for determining what constitutes a word. In order to be able to compare the results with the Reference Database (RDB) remember to use a sample 12 minutes in length from the total, 15-minute tape. Count all of the words that appear in each utterance, excluding only words appearing in mazes. Utterances with unintelligible segments and incomplete utterances are included in the count.

Miller (1991) has documented the following through statistical analysis of conversation and narrative transcripts of 257 children with normal language, three to 13 years of age:
• Each variable, MLU, NDW, and TNW is significantly correlated with age. While each can be argued to assess something independent about productive language: MLU–syntax, NDW–semantic diversity, TNW–overall verbal fluency, a composite measure of MLU, NDW, and TNW is the best predictor of age in both the conversation and narrative sampling conditions.
• The magnitude of the correlations is uniformly higher in the narrative condition suggesting that this condition is the best reflection of developmental change in general language skills through this period of development.
• The consistency of each variable in predicting age in the narrative condition suggests that each may be informative about the general development of different aspects of language production.

Differentiation of language disorders requires developmental measures to document overall productive language performance. The number of different words, total number of words, and mean length of utterance provide somewhat different indexes of language performance. With these measures, SLPs have the means to describe the relationship among linguistic levels at different points in development defining semantic diversity using NDW, syntax using MLU, and overall verbal productivity using TNW, or all three in combination. This strategy gives SLPs the opportunity to document different patterns of development where progress in language development is slower than expected for chronological age. Explanations for lower than expected mean length of utterance might include a syntactic deficit confirmed by a detailed, structural analysis or documentation of an oral motor control deficit which affects speech. Fewer different words than expected may be attributable to smaller vocabulary or retrieval problems. Fewer total words per unit time may be attributable to context, opportunity to talk, social-affective variables, or formulation deficits. Each of these conditions has a variety of potential explanations ranging from a lack of experience to storage deficits in short-term or long-term memory.

The three variables indexing developmental progress—MLU, NDW, TNW—are useful tools that document developmental delays or disordered performance. They will also help focus on specific aspects of language: semantic diversity, syntax, or overall productivity. The many uses of these variables will facilitate subsequent analyses to describe the specific nature of the problem in school-age children. These measures will provide an opportunity to document different patterns of language disorders, if they exist, by quantifying "error" patterns in language production relative to developmental level of language performance.

Measures of Disordered Performance

Measures of disordered performance are distinguished from measures of developmental progress. Measures of developmental progress correlate with age and measures of disordered performance quantify behaviors that interfere with communicative effectiveness. Experience has produced three categories of variables that can be interpreted as indicators of different types of disordered performance. They are mazes, speaking rate problems, and production errors.

Mazes

Mazes increase in narrative contexts, as compared to conversation, and also occur when longer utterances are attempted in both conversation and narrative contexts. The reference database documents maze frequency in both speaking contexts, providing reference information for children suspected of utterance formulation or word finding problems. Typically developing children produce a significant number of mazes in conversation and narrative samples. Children three to 13 years produce mazes in 15 to 25 percent of conversational samples and 20 to 41 percent of narrative samples.

The frequency of mazes increases with age, rather than decreases as one might expect. The mazes of typically developing children are usually limited to a single word or syllable, like "um" or "er," and are usually only one per utterance. Children with utterance formulation or word-finding problems usually produce longer mazes that are repetitions of the subject noun phrase. They may also be reformulations of the subject noun phrase, or noun phrase and part of the verb phrase, usually the auxiliary verb. For example, "The boy (The boy) was going to the mall" is a maze with a subject-noun phrase repetition, and "The boy (is, do) was going to the mall" is a maze with a verb-phrase reformulation. There are generally more than one maze per utterance for children with these problems.

Calculating Mazes

Mazes are marked by parenthesis at the time of transcription, noting false starts, "(do*) don/'t do that," repetitions, "(don/'t, don/'t), don/'t do that," and reformulations, "(I want, I won*) I don/'t do that." The use of (um), (er), or other such filled pauses are also marked as mazes. The distinction between a false start and a reformulation is vague at best and not particularly important for the initial analysis. At this level of analysis it is important to mark any material that is a repetition or revision of words or phrases that make up the body of the utterance. Count the number of utterances containing mazes. The initial analysis evaluates only the frequency of utterances that contain mazes. The RDB lists the corresponding mean and standard deviation of the child's peer group for the speaking condition. If this value exceeds one standard deviation, the SLP should follow-up with a more detailed analysis of the child's mazes. Mazes should be further analyzed when:

- the child produces a higher than expected frequency of utterances containing mazes,
- the mazes are unusually long,
- multiple mazes occur in single utterances, or
- the mazes significantly interfere with communication.

Look for the position of the mazes in utterances to note consistency; there may be a high proportion appearing before verb phrases. Also note the message the child is trying to express. The frequency of mazes may increase when the child attempts to express complex ideas concerning spatial, temporal, or causal relationships. This follow-up involves categorizing mazes by type and length. The categories are as follows:

- Filled Pauses:
— (um) The boy (er) went
- Repetitions:
— Part word: (Th*) The boy
— Word: (The) The boy
— Phrase: (The boy) The boy went . . .
- Revisions:
— Word: The (Boy) girl went . . .
— Phrase: (The girl is) The girl went . . .

Note that there are three major categories; filled pauses, repetitions, and revisions. SLPs generally can ignore the frequency of filled pauses since they rarely interfere with overall communication effectiveness. Revisions include both false starts and reformulations. There is general clinical agreement that revisions are more serious than repetitions and are generally associated with major word finding or utterance formulation deficits. The distinction between word finding and utterance formulation problems is signaled by the length of the unit of words involved in the maze. Children with word finding problems repeat part or whole words or revise single words. Children with utterance formulation problems produce a higher frequency of phrase repetitions and revisions relative to other maze types. The value of the analysis strategy is that it allows consideration of individual mazes where more than one maze may appear in an utterance. Children producing a high frequency of utterances with mazes are likely to produce more than one maze per utterance. It is not unusual for a child with a language disorder to produce 40 or more utterances with mazes and 80 or more individual mazes in a 100-utterance sample.

Speaking Rate Problems

Speaking rate problems are of two types: talking too fast or talking too slowly. Children who talk too fast threaten listeners with an overload of information before the listeners realize that though a child is talking at an incredible rate, he or she is failing to express much substantive content. Talking too slowly takes two forms: producing language at a consistently slow rate, with few words and utterances per unit of time; or pausing excessively between utterances which interrupts message flow and response expectation. SLPs should always allow more time for collecting language samples from children suspected of having language disorders for that reason. This lack of verbal productivity is a frustrating characteristic to listeners, yet researchers have not previously quantified it as a characteristic of language impairment. The rate data quantified in the 12-minute versions of the transcripts of the RDB (Appendix A) allow SLPs to compare an individual child's speaking rate in conversation and narrative speaking contexts with those of peers from the same age group.

Calculating Speaking Rate

The RDB contains several indicators of speaking rate, including the number of words and the number of utterances produced in samples 12 minutes long. If a sample is less than 12 minutes, the SLP can calculate the number of words (TNW) and the number of utterances per minute. The SLP should
- measure the duration of the sample by playing its taped version from start to finish and recording the exact length of time with a stopwatch, and
- enter the total time at the end of the transcript. For transcripts longer than 12 minutes, one simply reads the transcript while playing the tape with the stopwatch running, and
- stop at 12 minutes to mark the transcript.

When rate is a concern, the SLP or transcriber may want to mark the transcript at one minute intervals to note potential differences in the amount of talking during each consecutive minute. Count the total number of words in complete and intelligible utterances, and the number of complete and intelligible utterances the child produced in a 12-minute segment of the 15-minute taped sample. Compare these values with the child's peer group. When the transcript is shorter than 12 minutes, due to an inability to get a longer sample, count total words and utterances as specified for the 12-minute transcripts and divide each by the total duration of the transcript. The SLP may want to simplify this by counting words and utterances to the nearest minute. This calculation will provide the number of words and utterances produced per minute, which can then be compared with the Reference Database (RDB). Although it may be difficult to get a full 15 minutes from every child, SLPs should aim for that amount of time because it results in a more valid analysis of a representative 12 minutes.

Pauses

The pause is another variable. Pauses can occur between utterances or within an utterance. Research has shown that pauses of two seconds or longer are perceptible to the listener and usually signal that the speaker is willing to relinquish the floor, signalling a turn change. Children with certain language deficits appear to use pauses to search for the proper word or to gain adequate time to formulate an utterance. Several children, whose pause time totaled four to five minutes in a 15-minute sample, produced very few mazes. Apparently, the children paused until the utterance was formulated properly or the right word was found, then proceeded. Pauses or mazes may be different manifestations of the same long formulation problem though there is no research evidence yet to support this claim. Children who produce a significant number of pauses create very difficult pragmatic problems:
- How long does the listener wait before asking another question?
- Is the child failing to respond because she or he does not know the answer?
- Is she or he willfully avoiding a response to aggravate the listener?

- Is she or he unable to retrieve the proper word or formulate the response?

The SLP must approach each situation where a child exhibits a high frequency of pauses in the language sample with these questions and determine answers to them. The RDB provides several measures to quantify pausing difficulty, including the number of pauses within and between utterances, as well as total pause time for within and between utterance pauses.

Calculating Pauses

To calculate this measure the SLP needs only to mark the transcript when a pause greater than two seconds appears and count their overall occurrences. Children who produce a significant number of pauses require further analysis. To determine if the amount of elapsed time of the pauses is significantly greater than expected, the SLP will need to time each pause with a stopwatch. Add up the time of each pause to calculate pause time and compare it with the relevant peer group in the RDB. Pause data is significant for a number of children who seem to pause rather than "maze through" word or utterance formulation. Pauses should be considered as another variable documenting word finding or utterance formulation deficits.

Production Errors

Many production errors have potential diagnostic value. The analysis of these errors is a two-step process. First, the error must be identified at the time of transcription. These errors can be categorized into three frequently occurring types:

- Errors at the word level—overgeneralizations of irregular past tense verbs, pronoun errors, word choice errors, or failing to use specific reference when required.
- Errors at the utterance level—word order errors, coordination errors of tense or number.
- Content unclear errors—unclear semantic content or violated utterance contingency.

The transcriber codes these categories at the time of transcription to identify that a problem exists without analyzing its frequency.

Second, if the analysis of the transcript reveals high frequencies of these problems, the utterances must be grouped together for analysis. The task here is to search for commonalities among the words or utterances with errors. Consistent patterns of performance will lead to the identification of the child's disorder. Analyzing for developmentally appropriate errors becomes less of a concern as children get older, beginning around age seven. (Miller, 1981)

Omitting words or parts of words can be indicative of two types of problems: word finding problems or lack of knowledge of morpheme rules. There is little consistency in the literature regarding treatment of these behaviors because only a limited number of obligatory contexts can be identified. (Brown, 1973) Despite this situation, children with lexical deficits frequently omit words. What this means relative to the child's knowledge remains unclear.

Evaluating Production Errors

Assuming the transcriber has identified all utterances with errors, the SLP's task is to then evaluate these errors for potential insight into the nature of the child's language deficit. As a rule of thumb, unless more than ten percent of the child's utterances contain errors, further analysis will *not* be productive.

Begin the analysis by listing all the utterances with errors together, and review for commonalities such as a high number of either semantic, syntactic, or pragmatic errors. Do the same for utterances with word level errors. Formulate possible hypotheses to account for these errors, like word order violations or auxiliary verb errors involving numbers etc. Develop procedures to elicit further examples from the child to confirm the problem.

Other Measures of General Interest

Utterances per Speaking Turn

This measure is a simple count of the number of utterances each speaker produces per speaking turn. The measure will give an index of conversational samples. A distribution table can be helpful in identifying speaking partners who are dominating the conversation.

Figure 12

Child Turns	Number of Utterances	Adult Turns
8	1	7
6	2	5
4	3	8
2	4	9
1	5	7
0	6	5
0	7	3
0	8	2
0	9	0
0	10	0

Figure 12 indicates a child who has produced eight one-utterance turns, six two-utterance turns, and so on. The adult, however, is dominating the interaction with eight three-utterance turns, nine four-utterance turns, and so on. This adult is doing most of the talking in this conversation. Either the adult is pragmatically inappropriate with a domineering style, or the child is reticent, causing the adult to do more verbal prompting than would seem appropriate. The distribution of utterances per turn should be about equal in typical conversations.

Calculating Number of Utterances per Speaking Turn

Create a tally sheet with numbers one to ten. Review the entire transcript counting the number of utterances produced by each speaker per turn, recording each on the tally sheet. A turn is defined by the consecutive utterances produced by the same speaker or where utterances of the same speaker are separated by a pause marked by a ":" indicating a change in speaker turn. Appendix B contains the specific information about computer coding.

Frequency of Lexically Defined Grammatical Categories

The RDB provides the statewide normal language data to be used as a comparison with the reference sample. The relevant data to this category in the RDB are of two types, mean frequency of words and mean number of different words produced. These word lists can be diagnostic at a general level. The conjunctions, for example, provide a general index of utterance conjoining; the questions provide an index of question asking, as well as question type; and the negative list provides an index of negative utterance complexity. The questions and negatives provide frequency data on the production of these forms which will be useful if the SLP undertakes further syntactic analyses. If these forms are produced with low frequencies, an adequate sample may require additional sampling.

Counting Lexically Defined Grammatical Categories

In Appendix A, lists of questions, negatives, conjunctions, modals, and pronouns can be found with the accompanying frequency data. To use these lists to identify the words in each category in the transcript, count the number of times each word was produced and compare to the RDB data of the appropriate age and speaking condition.

Topic Maintenance and Change

Topic maintenance is essential for appropriate conversation. Knowing when to follow the same topic and when to change topics is a basic pragmatic skill. There are no precise ways to define topics when considering sequential utterances. An interesting conversation, for example, will include a mixture of new and old information. When SLPs try to use words to define the topic of an utterance they may not agree on the terms used. Most would agree on whether a specific utterance followed or changed the topic of the preceding utterance.

Coding Topic Maintenance and Change

Mark each utterance in the transcript as to topic maintenance (M) or topic change (C). This will produce a sequence of "M's" and "C's" that will allow quick inspection of maintenance and change behavior of the child relative to the examiner utterances.

Children who are having difficulty with topic maintenance exhibit one of two patterns: 1) Maintaining topic when following their own utterances, but changing topic following examiner utterances, or 2) changing topic for almost every utterance. It is common for topics to shift frequently at the beginning of a sample as speakers search for a mutually interesting topic. This analysis is very sensitive to social, affective, and pragmatic deficits.

Contingent Utterances

English usage has few forms requiring responses from listeners, but those which exist can be grouped usefully under the heading of contingent forms. These include the following:

Figure 13

Contingent Utterance Forms

Comment:	"I'm going to the store."
and	
Acknowledgement:	"OK"
Comment:	"I'm going to the store."
and	
Contingent Query:	"The store?"
Contingent Query:	"The store?"
and	
Response:	"Yes"
Request:	"Why are you going to the store?"
and	
Response:	"To get some milk"
Directive:	"Go to the store."
and	
Compliance:	"OK"

Coding Contingent Utterances

First, locate the contingent utterance combinations in the sample and then code the response utterances for appropriate or inappropriate response to the contingency. If the child has more than ten percent inappropriate utterances in contingent contexts, evaluate the extent to which this behavior interferes with communicative effectiveness. This analysis will confirm or negate inappropriate responses.

Repair and Revisions

Children must learn to request clarification when they do not understand the utterance of the speaking partner. They must also alter their productions to provide clarification when requested. Children with language disorders have been reported to have difficulty with both of these aspects of conversation.

Coding Repairs and Revisions

Identify all of the requests for clarification. Evaluate the responses for appropriateness and form. Initially, young children will respond to requests for clarification by simply repeating the initial utterance; when pressed they will repeat, only louder. As children get older, they can better determine the part of the utterance with which the listener was having difficulty and provide the necessary information. There should be evidence of sensitivity on the part of the child that she or he is not being understood. If the sensitivity does not appear, then a pragmatic problem may exist.

Loban Analysis

A detailed description of Loban's analysis procedure can be found in Appendix C. This analysis provides an easy way to check general developmental progress using the mean length of communication unit measure, general structural complexity using the proportion of utterances with dependent clauses measure, and the frequency and density of mazes. These measures are calculated on 30 communication units produced in a narrative context. Loban defined a communication unit as an independent clause with any associated dependent clauses. He presents data on these measures by grade level for children in K-12. The relatively few number of utterances and the two-year age range for each grade category limit the use of this measure for exploration. It will be useful for identifying children who require further LSA analysis because of frequent mazes or short simple utterances predominating their speech. The Loban analysis is complimentary to other general analyses presented here. Keep in mind that if one calculates a Loban analysis for every 30 utterances, in a 100-utterance sample different results may occur across analyses. Thirty utterances is not enough to produce a stable analysis.

The Advantages of Computer-Aided Analysis

Costs and Benefits

Computer-assisted analysis systems have been in use since the early 1960's on mainframe computers. Initially, research laboratories developed these systems to relieve the labor intensive process of transcribing and coding children's conversations with their parents, allowing investigators to quantify developmental progress. More recent approaches have evolved with the availability of personal computers, making computer solutions accessible outside the laboratory. A variety of computer solutions are now available within public school settings to help SLPs complete required job responsibilities in a more time-efficient manner. Some of these tasks include generation of reports, IEPs, scheduling, and now, interpretation of language samples.

Computer technology for LSA is beneficial at all levels: transcription, analysis, and interpretation. At the transcription level, computers require a standard format to recognize the word, morpheme, and utterance for analysis. The consistency of this transcription format therefore results in greater reliability because decision rules are clearly articulated. A format-error-checking routine within the computer program assures accuracy of the transcript format. Error-checking also helps SLPs avoid computational errors. Failing to include terminal punctuation on an utterance could cause it to be treated as part of the following utterance resulting in an inflated MLU. The standard transcription format used in computer programs improves reliability and accuracy as well as the ability to share transcripts and the resultant analyses and interpretation. Readability is another important benefit provided by computerized LSA. The benefits of insisting on a readable transcript format using standard English facilitates the sharing of information with parents and teachers.

There are several other distinct advantages that computers offer for performing language sample analyses.

- Speed: Computers can perform in seconds analyses that would take hours by hand.
- Accuracy: Computers perform endless counts, sorts, and calculations without error.
- Variety: Computers make it possible to perform multiple analyses on the same transcript like different linguistic levels and/or multiple transcripts in succession. These benefits result in more analyses being performed per unit of time, making much more data available to the SLP for interpretation.

The greatest benefit of computer LSA is the interpretation of individual performance. The standardization of transcription and the increased number of analyses allow the SLP to compare a child's performance across linguistic units, as well as compare performance between children. These standard methodologies have allowed Wisconsin to develop a database of performance across ages for standard speaking conditions. Through the use of this database the SLP now has the ability to compare the performance of the referred child with Wisconsin peers. The use of this database will lead to improved accuracy in identifying children with language deficits as well as extend understanding of normal developmental progress. LSA also enhances the SLP's credibility because it can support, quantitatively, the progress of children in therapy, monitoring and documenting their problems and growth on a yearly basis more expeditiously than analysis done by hand. It is apparent that computers offer a number of significant advantages which doing LSA by hand cannot match.

The computer systems and software must be learned in order to make them work. The opportunities offered by computer-aided LSA require rethinking measurement, interpretation, and constitution of disordered performance. It is this last area that is difficult to document, but is probably the most important for implementing computer-aided LSA. In determining a language disordered performance, the SLP must consider several areas: the rules the computer uses for the calculations performed; the relationship between the level of detail included in the transcript and the resultant analyses; and the relationship among levels and units of analysis. Clearly, computer-aided LSA increases the demand for knowledge about computers, language development, and language disorders. The demand for more expertise in using computers and specific software in LSA requires inservice training.

Language Sample Analysis Software

Two approaches have emerged in designing software for LSA. The first is the dedicated analysis approach, where the program is designed to perform a specific analysis or set of analyses. Examples of this type would be Lingquest 1 (Mordecai, Palin, and Palmer, 1985), Automated LARSP (Language Assessment, Remediation, and Screening Procedure) (Bishop, 1985), or Computerized Profiling. (Long and Fey, 1989) The second approach offers the user unlimited coding and analysis options by providing both standard pre-configured analysis and user-designed analyses. Examples of this approach are SALT: Systematic Analysis of Language Transcripts (Miller and Chapman, 1991), and PAL: Pye Analysis of Language. (Pye, 1987) See Figure 14 for a listing of several computer programs that perform LSA.

■ Figure 14

Computer Programs that Perform LSA	
Dedicated Analysis	**Unlimited Coding**

Automated LARSP
    (Bishop, 1985)
Computerized Profiling
    (Long and Fey, 1989)
DSS Computer Program
    (Hixson, 1983)
Lingquest I
    (Mordecai, Palin, and Palmer, 1985)
Parrot Easy Language Sample Analysis
(PELSA)
    (Weiner, 1988)
	Child Language Data Exchange
	System (CHILDES)
	    (MacWhinney and Snow, 1991)
	Pye Analysis of Language (PAL)
	    (Pye, 1987)
	Systematic Analysis of Language
	Transcripts (SALT)
	    (Miller and Chapman, 1991)

Programs of the first type have computer versions of analyses developed and reported in the literature of the field to document developmental progress of specific language levels, for instance, syntax. In fact most of these programs, most notably LARSP and DSS, perform various syntactic analyses. Computerized Profiling performs standard analysis at three linguistic levels: syntax, semantic, and pragmatic. These analyses describe developmental progress at each of these linguistic levels. The focus of programs like Computerized Profiling, LARSP, DSS, PRISM, and CAP document developmental knowledge and characterize disordered performance as limited syntactic, semantic or pragmatic frequency, diversity, or complexity. Each of these analyses covers a specific period of development usually five to seven years of age.

There are several limitations to these measures. Most notable is the lack of data (normative or criterion reference) with which to interpret any individual child's performance. There is also no evidence documenting that any of these measures are sensitive to description of language disorder, beyond documenting developmental progress. Nonetheless, these measures can be informative, particularly the syntactic analyses, in providing a formal description of structural complexity.

The computer-assisted LSA tool which provided the basis for the RDB is SALT. SALT was developed by Dr. Jon Miller and Dr. Robin Chapman, University of Wisconsin-Madison, as a means of analyzing the communicative attempts of one or more speakers during an interaction. The SALT program provides detailed interactive analysis of free speech samples from one or more speakers. These programs have been designed to provide SLPs with powerful language analysis tools to meet individual diagnostic and program evaluation needs.

Resources for Detailed Analyses

This section has provided the strategy of using general analyses as an index of problems as well as an indicator of developmental progress, error patterns, and communicative effectiveness. More complex, detailed analysis of these areas at all language levels will be required in order to document the nature of some children's language deficit. Therefore, Figure 15 lists resources and references so SLPs will be able to locate appropriate materials as needed. Figure 15 lists the major analyses that have been used over the past 15 years to analyze various aspects of productive language. Note that most of them deal with syntax, though more recent work has added many important analyses of pragmatic performance. The most useful of these for identifying specific pragmatic deficits is the Prutting and Kirchner (1987) analysis. See Appendix D, Resources, for more detailed information on appropriate materials.

■ Figure 15

Resources for the Detailed Analysis of Language Samples

Content	Procedure	Age Range
Syntax	Developmental Sentence Scoring (DSS) (Lee, 1974)	3 - 7 years
	Language Assessment Remediation and Screening Procedure (LARSP) (Crystal, Fletcher, and Garman, 1976)	2 - 5 years
	Assigning Structural Stage (ASS) (Miller, 1981)	18 months - 7 years
Semantics	Semantic relations expressed in conjunctions (Miller, 1981)	29 months - 10 years
	Semantic information requested by question forms (Miller, 1981)	18 months - 8 years
	Semantic relations expressed by verbal predicates (Johnston, 1981)	18 months - 7 years
Syntax/Semantics Combined	Phase (Bloom and Lahey, 1978; Lahey, 1987)	8 months - 8 years
Pragmatics	Intentional analysis (Chapman, 1981)	8 months - 5 years
	Story grammar	3 years - adult
	Social routines Pragmatic Protocol (Prutting and Kirchner, 1987)	8 months - adult

The resources outlined here considers the information provided by the general analyses across areas to identify performance problems. All of these measures can be calculated using paper and pencil. However, a computer will be able to calculate measures of developmental progress and error analyses in seconds. With additional coding, many detailed analyses (see Figure 15) can be calculated in a time-efficient manner. Analysis done by hand will limit the SLP's time, type of analysis, and accuracy. The guide has outlined procedures for hand analysis to provide an explicit account of the calculation of each variable. These calculation methods are the same as those used by SALT in deriving the scores for these same general measures. This consistency makes the RDB data useful for interpretation regardless of the method of calculation. Please see Appendix F for more information on cost-effectiveness of LSA.

References

Bishop, D. *Automated LARSP*. Computer software. Manchester, England: University of Manchester, 1985.

Bloom, L., and M. Lahey. *Language Development and Language Disorders*. New York: Wiley, 1978.

Brown, R. *A First Language*. Cambridge, MA: Harvard University Press, 1973.

Chapman, R. "Exploring Children's Communicative Intents." In *Assessing Language Production in Children: Experimental Procedures*. Ed. J. Miller. Austin, TX: PRO-ED, 1981, pp. 111-138.

Crystal, D., P. Fletcher, and M. Garman. *The Grammatical Analysis of Language Disability: A Procedure for Assessment and Remediation*. The Hague: Elsevier-North Holland Publishing Co., 1976. (The second, 1991 edition is now available through the Singular Publishing Group, Inc. of San Diego.)

Hixson, P. *Developmental Sentence Scoring*. Computer software. Omaha, NE: Computer Language Analysis, 1983.

Johnston, J. "A Computer Program for the Automated Analysis of English Predicates." Unpublished procedure. Vancouver, BC: Department of Speech and Hearing Sciences, University of British Columbia, 1991.

Kent, R. "Anatomical and Neuromuscular Maturation of the Speech Mechanism: Evidence from Acoustic Studies." *Journal of Speech and Hearing Research* 19 (1976), pp. 421-445.

Kent, R. "Psychobiology of Speech Development: Coemergence of Language and the Movement System." *American Journal of Physiology* 25 (1984), pp. 888-894.

Klee, T., et al. "A Comparison of the Age-MLU Relation in Normal and Specifically Language Impaired Preschool Children." *Journal of Speech and Hearing Disorders* 54 (1989), pp. 226-233.

Lahey, M. *Language Disorders and Language Development*. New York: MacMillan Publishing Co., 1987.

Lee, L. *Developmental Sentence Analysis*. Evanston, IL: Northwestern University Press, 1974.

Loban, W. *Language Development: Kindergarten Through Grade Twelve*. Research report No. 18. Urbana, IL: National Council of Teachers of English, 1976.

Long, S., and M. Fey. *Computerized Language Profiling Version 6.1*. Computer software. Ithaca, NY: Ithaca College, 1989.

MacWinney, B., and C. Snow. "The Child Language Data Exchange System" (CHILDES). Computer software. Pittsburgh, PA: Carnegie-Mellon University, 1991.

Miller, J. "Quantifying Productive Language Disorder." In *Research on Child Language Disorders: A Decade of Progress*. Ed. J. Miller. Austin, TX: PRO-ED, 1991, pp. 211-220.

Miller, J. *The Reference Database Project*. Madison, WI: Language Analysis Laboratory, Waisman Center, University of Wisconsin, 1990.

Miller, J. F. *Assessing Language Production in Children: Experimental Procedures*. Austin, TX: PRO-ED, 1981.

Miller J., and R. Chapman. *SALT: A computer program for the Systematic Analysis of Language Transcripts*. Computer software. Madison, WI: University of Wisconsin, 1991.

Mordecai, D., M. Palin, and C. Palmer. *Lingquest 1*. Computer software. Columbus, OH: Charles E. Merrill, 1985.

Prutting, C., and D. Kirchner. "A Clinical Appraisal of the Pragmatic Aspects of Language." *Journal of Speech and Hearing Disorders* 52 (1987), pp. 99-104.

Pye, C. *Analysis of Language*. Computer software. Lawrence, KS: University of Kansas, 1987.

Weiner, P. "The Value of Follow-up Studies." *Topics in Language Disorders* 5.3 (June, 1985), pp. 78-92.

5

Interpretation

Using the Reference Database

Sections 1 through 4 have discussed the methods and procedures required to document productive language performance using Language Sample Analysis. The data derived from this methodology are extensive and require organization for interpretation because of the diverse types of problems exhibited by children with language disorders. The first step in interpretation is distinguishing essentially normal from disordered performance. Secondly, SLPs must also distinguish delays in productive language development from productive language disorders. Finally, the SLP must identify and document the specific areas of deficit requiring further analysis, and then develop an intervention plan.

A basic tool for interpreting language performance is the RDB which provides the performance data from children with typically developing language. The RDB contains summary information derived from transcripts of 266 children ages three through 13 years. The data are organized by age, with separate data reported for ages three, four, five, six, seven, nine, 11, and 13. These data, in Appendix A, are organized by the two major speaking conditions—conversation and narration—and by the length of the transcript used for the analyses—100 complete and intelligible utterances or 12 minutes in duration. The data provide the information necessary to determine if the performance of a specific child is within or outside of the expected range for typically developing children on a variety of measures.

The first section of the RDB is divided into information about the conversational and narrative content and rate summaries. The following page (the Content and Rate Summary of Conversation for Five-year-olds) is taken directly from the RDB. This section of the RDB contains one page of summary information on 24 content variables, such as MLU, Type Token Ratio, Total Words, etc., based on 100 complete and intelligible utterances. The page also includes 11 rate variables, Total Utterances, Complete and Intelligible Utterances, and Total Words, etc., based on a 12-minute version of the total transcript. There is a total of 35 variables for each age and speaking condition. The variables are listed on the left from top to bottom, beginning with MLU. Horizontally, the numerical values move from left to right and begin with the mean group performance: (5.71); the standard deviation (0.91); the performance range of one standard deviation plus or minus from the mean (4.81 - 6.62); the percent standard deviation (16 percent); and the range (four to seven).

Following all of the Content and Rate summaries in the RDB (Appendix A) is one page containing two distributional tables with the mean percentage of utterances with mazes at each utterance length for conversation and narrative samples. The final section of the RDB contains word list summaries organized by age group and speaking condition. The word list summaries provide statistics for several word categories of syntactic and semantic interest; such as questions, conjunctions, negatives, modals, and pronouns. Data are provided for each word in the word lists. The RDB provides sufficient data to determine if the performance of a student in any specific analyses is within the expected range of performance for children of the same age and speaking condition.

These descriptive statistics should provide the information necessary to interpret individual scores relative to the reference sample. Keep in mind that these are not "norms," but criterion data, documenting performance of children from Wisconsin where samples were collected, transcribed, and analyzed under similar conditions.

Figure 16

Content and Rate Summary / 5-Year-Olds

(Conversation N=28)

	Content						
	100 Utterance Samples						
Variables	**Mean**	**SD**	**SD–**	**SD+**	**%SD**	**R–**	**R+**
Mean Length of Utterance (MLU)	5.71	0.91	4.81	6.62	16%	4	7
Type Token Ratio	0.45	0.05	0.40	0.50	11%	0	1
Total Words	520	81	439	602	16%	380	645
Different Words	181	25	156	206	14%	117	228
Utterances with Mazes	22	9	13	31	42%	7	40
Utterances with Overlaps	11	6	6	17	49%	0	22
Bound Morphemes Frequency							
Regular Past	4	3	1	6	75%	0	10
Plural	15	8	7	22	51%	2	31
Possessive	2	2	0	5	102%	0	9
Third Person Singular	7	5	2	11	73%	1	23
Present Progressive	5	4	1	8	73%	0	16
Utterance Content							
Personal Pronouns (Total)	81	15	67	96	18%	55	110
(Types)	10	1	8	11	15%	6	12
Total Questions	7	6	1	13	81%	0	22
(WH Total)	4	4	0	8	89%	0	15
(WH Types)	2	1	1	3	56%	0	4
Negatives (Total)	13	5	7	18	41%	4	23
(Types)	5	1	4	7	27%	3	8
Conjunctions (Total)	42	18	24	60	43%	11	76
(Types)	7	1	5	8	20%	4	10
Modals (Total)	6	4	2	10	72%	0	14
(Types)	2	1	1	4	51%	0	5

	Rate						
	12 Minute Samples						
Variables	**Mean**	**SD**	**SD–**	**SD+**	**%SD**	**R–**	**R+**
Total Utterances	149	27	123	176	18%	108	211
Complete and Intelligible Utterances	139	27	112	166	19%	99	193
Total Words	724	187	537	911	26%	423	1140
Different Words	219	39	179	258	18%	144	315
Mean Length of Utterance (MLU)	5.71	0.87	4.84	6.58	15%	4	7
Between Utterance Pauses	21.61	12.54	9.07	34.15	58%	4	49
Between Utterance Pause Time	1.26	0.86	0.40	2.12	68%	0.2	3.6
Within Utterance Pauses	2.43	2.96	-0.53	5.39	122%	0	10
Within Utterance Pause Time	0.15	0.21	-0.05	0.36	135%	0.0	0.7
Words per Minute	69.48	17.69	51.79	87.18	25%	40	105
Utterances per Minute	12.48	2.24	10.23	14.72	18%	9	18

The critical feature for documenting language disorder is the criteria for normal performance. In previous sections, one standard deviation and below has been used to identify performances that are of concern, and therefore require follow-up analysis. Usually, a performance that is one standard deviation above or below the mean is *not* significant enough to warrant identification of the student as language disordered. SLPs must differentiate problem areas from handicapping conditions when determining an Exceptional Educational Need (EEN). SLPs must remember that one standard deviation should not be considered the criteria for determining disordered performance.

There is no statewide measure mandating the specific degree of deficit (in terms of standard deviation units) required to indicate a handicapping condition and a need for special education. Most multi-disciplinary teams make these decisions using parameters ranging from minus one and one-half to two standard deviations from the mean. The M-team makes these decisions in conjunction with its knowledge of how the student's disorder interferes with his or her ability to acquire and utilize knowledge, maintain satisfactory social relationships, or have sound emotional development. The Reference Database allows districts to employ, for the first time, the same performance standards in LSA as in standardized tests. Using the data in Figure 16, for example, an MLU between 4.81 and 6.62 would be considered to be within the expected performance range for five-year-old children. An MLU below 4.81 would be considered a problem, and the child's performance on other variables would need to be evaluated. The issue of the type of deficit can then be addressed systematically to determine the specific nature of the disordered performance, if any exists.

Summarizing Assessment Data

There are a number of ways to summarize the information obtained through LSA. One way is to organize the data in terms of measurements of delay (MLU, Number of Different Words, Total Words), and measurements of disorder (Mazes, Abandoned Utterances, Errors at the Word or Utterance Level, etc.). Another way is to incorporate the same numerical information into a framework of linguistic categories such as semantics, syntax, and pragmatics. SLPs in the Madison Metropolitan School District found that a framework which combined both methods is the most informative and comprehensive. (See Figure 17.)

Figure 17

LSA Summary Form (blank)

Conversation or Narration _____

Comparison to _____-Year-Olds

Student Name _____   Age _____

File Name _____

Examiner _____

Date of Sample _____

Measure	Student	Mean	SD	SD–	SD+	%SD	R–	R+	Comments
I. Timing (12 Minute Data)									
Total Utterances	—								
Complete and Intelligible Utterances	—								
Between Utterance Pauses	—								
Between Utterance Pause Time	—								
Within Utterance Pauses	—								
Within Utterance Pause Time	—								
Number of Utterances per Minute	—								
Number of Words per Minute	—								
Final Timing	—								
II. Intelligibility (100 Utterance Data)									
Percentage of Complete and Intelligible Utterances	—								
III. Mazes and Overlaps (100 Utterance Data)									
Utterances w/Mazes	—								
Filled Pauses ("um")	—								
Repetitions									
— Part Word	—								
— Word	—								
— Phrase	—								
Revisions									
— Word	—								
— Phrase	—								
Utterances w/Overlaps	—								
Also See Timing Information									

Measure	Student	Mean	SD	SD-	SD+	%SD	R-	R+	Comments
IV. Semantics (100 Utterance Data)									
Type Token Ratio	___								
Total Words	___								
Different Words	___								
V. Word Lists (100 Utterance Data)									
(Total) Questions: How, What, When, Where, Which, Who, Whose, Why									
Negatives: Ain't, Are/n't, Can/'t, Could/n't, Did/n't, Does/n't, Don't, Had/n't, Has/n't, Have/n't, Is/n't, Might/n't, Must/n't, No, Nope, Not, Should/n't, Uhuh, Was/n't, Were/n't, Won't, Would/n't									
(Total)	___								
(Types)	___								
Conjunctions: After, And, As, Because, But, If, Or, Since, So, Then, Until, While									
(Total)	___								
(Types)	___								
Modals: Can, Could, May, Might, Must, Shall, Should, Will, Would									
(Total)	___								
(Types)	___								
Personal Pronouns: He, Her, Him, I, It, Me, She, Them, They, Us, We, You									
(Total)	___								
(Types)	___								
VI. Syntax/Morphology (100 Utterance Data)									
MLU-Morphemes	___								
VII. Bound Morphemes (100 Utterance Data)									
Third Person Singular (/3S)	___								
Regular Past (/ED)	___								
Present Progressive (/ING)	___								
Plural (/S)	___								
Possessive (/Z)	___								
Also See Word Lists									

Levels of Error Analysis

Morpheme Level:

EO: _____ Occurrences

Word Level:

EW: _____ Occurrences (Include both semantic and syntactic errors.)

Pronoun Error:

EP: _____ Occurrences

Sentence and Discourse Levels:

EU: _____ Occurrences

CU: _____ Occurrences

How confident are you that this sample represents
a true picture of the student's language skills?   Unsure 1 2 3 4 5 6 7 Very Confident

How confident are you that the topics discussed
were familiar and comfortable to the student?   Unsure 1 2 3 4 5 6 7 Very Confident

Is the language behavior documented in this sample
observed in other settings and with other speaking
partners?   ☐ Yes ☐ No

How do the problems identified in the sample handicap the student in his/her educational environment?

59

This form shows the categories used by these SLPs from MMSD to take the information provided by SALT or from hand analyses and summarize it in a way that is clinically relevant and easy to use. The LSA Summary Form incorporates both more traditional ways of thinking about language (Intelligibility, Semantics, Syntax/Morphology) and the organizational framework suggested by the research documented in this volume (data describing language disorder like rate and timing, mazes, overlaps, and error categories) and incorporates both in a single format.

Once the data from the language sample are organized and tabulated on the summary form, the SLP must refer to the reference database for the statistics which help to interpret the student's performance. The SLP writes the values representing the mean, standard deviation, percentage of standard deviation (%SD), and range of performance for the comparison group from the reference database on the summary form. The standard deviations, above or below the mean (SD+/SD−), are calculated by adding or subtracting one or more standard deviations from the mean. When complete, the student's performance can be compared directly to the mean performance of the appropriate age group and for the appropriate speaking condition. The clinician makes note of any value that is significantly discrepant in the far right-hand column for later interpretation. This strategy is encouraged for SLPs who are beginning to use and interpret data from LSA. With experience, SLPs may find that they wish to customize this summary format to meet their personal needs better. *Summary forms complete with data for each age and speaking condition from the RDB will be available during LSA training.*

Summarizing the results of each analysis according to the feature of language performance it quantifies will bring the data into focus for each child, documenting strengths and weaknesses of the child's language performance. This process can be tedious given the number of variables that should be analyzed in order to document the range of performance variables. A computer program has recently been completed that compiles this type of summary automatically, comparing the individual child to the Reference Database. This program, SALT Database Profiler, has been designed as a companion to SALT, to provide SLPs with a standard summary of general analyses at the word and utterance level. This program automatically identifies those variables that are one or two standard deviations above or below the mean. A second level of analyses is available to examine more carefully those variables outside one standard deviation of the Reference Database. Maze analyses at this level, for example, are categorized and counted as filled pauses, repetitions, or revisions, by length, at the part-word, word, or phrase level. A variety of maze distribution tables are provided as well. Finally the program provides a third level of analysis by providing access to several types of utterances that may require more detailed analyses, like utterances with errors. Keep in mind that these summaries are of general analyses. The data provided may be sufficient for identification of disordered status, but more detailed analyses may be required in some cases to develop sufficient description for an appropriate intervention plan. This is particularly the case for pragmatic or discourse level problems.

Putting It All Together

Section 1 of this guide presented information regarding the six most common types of productive language disorders on SLPs' caseloads. Training supported by the Department of Public Instruction will use examples of each type to provide practice for SLPs in the interpretation of data obtained from LSA. (See Appendix G for case studies of each type for review.)

This section will take a single student and SLP scenario and go sequentially through the decision-making process to illustrate simply how to use LSA in identification and programming of a student with a language disorder. At the end of this section, Figure 19 offers an overall checklist of the steps to follow when using LSA.

A Case Study

Before collecting the sample, the SLP checked the recording equipment. The recorder had been cleaned recently and an external microphone was available. Although the room was sometimes noisy when classes were in the hall, the SLP planned to collect the sample in between these times. In addition, other ambient noise was reduced as much as possible to provide a good quality recording. While checking the recording equipment, the SLP put the student's name, age, date, and the type of sample to be collected both on the audio track and on the tape label for later reference. The age of this student is eight years.

The language sample was collected as part of an M-team re-evaluation. The child had been receiving speech and language therapy since he was referred to the public schools at two and one-half years of age because of an expressive language disorder and poor articulation. Academic difficulties in reading were also of concern to the parent who requested the evaluation. There were no other academic or social problems. Learning disabilities and speech and language were suspected handicapping conditions.

The SLP planned to collect a conversational language sample and decided to use the child's recent dinner out at Ginza, a local Japanese restaurant, for their interaction. She jotted down several additional questions and topics including other favorite restaurants and foods to use if the conversation did not move along smoothly.

She used the sampling protocol from Section 2 as a guide in developing her questions. Because of her familiarity with the child, she knew no other materials would be required.

When he arrived in the therapy room, the SLP made the child comfortable. They talked briefly about other matters and then she explained the task for the day. She showed him how the tape recorder worked and promised that he could listen to the tape later. They discussed the kinds of questions she would ask and laid out the timeline for collecting the sample.

They conversed naturally for about 15 minutes. The SLP followed the child's lead and introduced the new topics she had planned only when needed to keep the conversation going. When they were finished, the tape was rewound and they listened to part of it together. This allowed the SLP to check the tape quality and to make notes that would clarify content later during the transcription process. It also helped to confirm that the sample was typical of the child's usual language production. The tape was transcribed using standard conventions which are summarized in Appendix B.

Transcript of a Conversational Language Sample
The following is an excerpt from the transcript:

    1   E   So what kind/s of thing/s do you get to eat there at Ginza?
    2   C   Well I only (I) went there once (and the) and I ate chicken.
    3   C   (Um what) what/'re those like uncleben thing/s?
    4   E   Rice?
    5   C   Yeah rice and we put some stuff on it what [EW:that]
    6   taste good [EU].

7	C	And the chicken too.
8	C	We put everything on it and I don't know what a [EW:the]
9		other stuff is called.
10	E	It was good though, huh?
11	C	Yes.
12	E	Great!
13	C	And they give [EW:gave] us the [EW:a] show. {Tense: is this past or
14		present?}
15	C	They'll go like {boo boo boo boo} for a little.
16	C	(They'll ju*) juggle/ing (um) the pepper shaker (and the salt sha*)
17		and (sh*) salt.
18	E	Do they juggle anything else?
19	C	(N*) no, (they throw) if you have (um) shrimp they'll throw the
20		(um) crab thing/s [CU].
21	C	You know what.
22	C	The pincher thing/s.
23	E	Uhhuh.
24	C	They'll throw it [EW:them] at (me) people.
25	C	And they throw (um)>
26	C	(At our) when I went they throw [EW:threw] (um)>
27	C	What you know call it [EU].
28	C	Yes, (um) you know what/'s in>
29	C	Oh yeah, (san*) pepper shaker, a different kind [CU].
30	C	And my sister never went there, but my mom and my dad and me
31		[EW:I] went there.
32	C	And my sister/'s the only one who (have/n't) has not (g*) went
33		[EW:gone] there.

The SLP then analyzed the transcript using the SALT program, but the same information could have been obtained using the hand analyses summarized in Section 4.

The SLP took the data provided by SALT and entered it on a summary form to help her analyze and interpret the student's performance. She selected the summary form for nine-year-olds since she knew that the child was of at least average cognitive ability. This was later confirmed by the psychologist. Figure 18 shows a completed summary form for this child.

Figure 18

LSA Summary Form (completed)

Conversation
Comparison to Nine-Year-Olds

Student Name _____   Examiner _____
File Name _____   Date of Sample _____

Age __8-0__

Measure	Student	Mean	SD	SD–	SD+	%SD	R–	R+	Comments
I. Timing (12 Minute Data)									
Total Utterances	110	181	31	150	212	17%	104	249	Note: Final timing for 100 utterances was 8 min. 24 sec. Thus student values should be about 75% of the mean.
Complete and Intelligible Utterances	100	167	29	138	197	17%	84	233	
Between Utterance Pauses	1	7.70	6.35	1.35	14.06	82%	0	25	
Between Utterance Pause Time	:03	0.40	0.44	-0.04	0.83	110%	0.0	2.1	
Within Utterance Pauses	2	1.67	1.82	-0.15	3.49	109%	0	6	
Within Utterance Pause Time	:05	0.08	0.09	-0.01	0.17	109%	0.0	0.3	
Number of Utterances per Minute	13.10	15.11	2.59	12.52	17.70	17%	9	21	
Number of Words per Minute	82.38	96.12	25.10	71.02	121.22	26%	40	146	
Final Timing	8.24	12	0	12	12	0%	12	12	all ok
II. Intelligibility (100 Utterance Data)									
Percentage of Complete and Intelligible Utterances	91.82	92.35	4.53	87.83	96.88	5%	80.65	99.01	Sounds immature
III. Mazes and Overlaps (100 Utterance Data)									
Utterances w/Mazes	34 (卌 IIII)	23	7	16	30	32%	8	39	*between /and 1½ SD above the mean
Filled Pauses ("um")	卌 IIII	9							
Repetitions									
— Part Word	卌 II 7 }16								
— Word	IIII 4 }								
— Phrase	卌 5 }								
Revisions									
— Word	卌 II								
— Phrase	卌 卌 卌 卌 卌 20 }21								
Utterances w/Overlaps	11 (10%)	0	0	0	0	0%	0	0	
Also See Timing Information									

Comments (handwritten):
- revises pronouns, eg. (we) I'm gonna have...
- starts one word and abandons, eg. (sh*) salt (g*) went.
- overlaps are disconcerting to conversational partner

Measure	Student	Mean	SD	SD−	SD+	%SD	R−	R+	Comments
IV. Semantics (100 Utterance Data)									
Type Token Ratio	.41	0.44	0.06	0.38	0.50	14%	0	1	ok
Total Words	651	592	95	496	687	16%	431	742	ok
Different Words	208	209	26	183	235	13%	167	278	ok
V. Word Lists (100 Utterance Data)									
(Total) Questions: How, What, When, Where, Which, Who, Whose, Why	1	2	2	-1	4	127%	0	8	
Negatives: Ain't, Are/n't, Can't, Could/n't, Did/n't, Does/n't, Don't, Had/n't, Has/n't, Have/n't, Is/n't, Might/n't, Must/n't, No, Nope, Not, Should/n't, Uhuh, Was/n't, Were/n't, Won't, Would/n't									
(Total)	21	11	6	5	17	53%	1	25	
(Types)	6	5	2	3	7	42%	1	10	
Conjunctions: After, And, As, Because, But, If, Or, Since, So, Then, Until, While									
(Total)	62	61	23	39	84	37%	27	112	
(Types)	7	8	1	6	9	15%	6	10	
Modals: Can, Could, May, Might, Must, Shall, Should, Will, Would									
(Total)	8	4	2	2	6	58%	0	9	
(Types)	5	2	1	1	3	48%	0	4	
Personal Pronouns: He, Her, Him, I, It, Me, She, Them, They, Us, We, You									
(Total)	95	85	16	69	101	19%	41	117	
(Types)	11	9	1	8	11	14%	6	12	
VI. Syntax/Morphology (100 Utterance Data)									
MLU-Morphemes	7.25	6.50	1.06	5.44	7.56	16%	5	8	Post-V
VII. Bound Morphemes (100 Utterance Data)									
Third Person Singular (/3S)	8	6	3	2	9	59%	0	15	
Regular Past (/ED)	2/3	4	3	1	8	74%	0	16	Omitted /ed once
Present Progressive (/ING)	2	4	3	2	7	60%	0	10	
Plural (/S)	17	20	8	11	28	43%	5	44	
Possessive (/Z)	3	3	2	0	5	94%	0	12	
Also See Word Lists									

Spontaneous language contains frequent overgeneralization of past tense → buyed/bought, goed/went

*also frequently uses non-specific words like "stuff"

Levels of Error Analysis

Morpheme Level:

EO: **1**   Occurrences

#273 watch/watched

Word Level: 9

EW: Occurrences (Include both semantic and syntactic errors.)

#71 from/for   #152 couldn't/can't   #172 give/gave, the/a
#18 of/for   #163 what/that   #185 throw/threw
   #167 a/the   #192 went/gone

Pronoun Error: 3

EP: Occurrences

#190 me/I
#183 it/them
#105 all/every

Sentence and Discourse Levels:

EU: **10**   Occurrences

#49   #102   #163   #256
#74   #123   #166
#77   #128   #228

CU (content unclear) often reflects word finding difficulties.

CU: **11**   Occurrences

#71   #141   #148   #188   #232
#102   #143   #179   #204   #241
   #206

How confident are you that this sample represents
a true picture of the student's language skills?   Unsure 1 2 3 4 5 6 ⑦ Very Confident

How confident are you that the topics discussed
were familiar and comfortable to the student?   Unsure 1 2 3 4 5 6 ⑦ Very Confident

Is the language behavior documented in this sample
observed in other settings and with other speaking
partners?   ☒ Yes ☐ No

How do the problems identified in the sample handicap the student in his/her educational environment?

Adults don't always know what he is talking about.
Reading difficulties may be related to word finding.
Uses rising intonation frequently; strings many utterances together
so that the listener is unsure of what he is saying.

Looking at the first section, Timing, the SLP noted that all values were within one standard deviation of the nine-year-olds in the Reference Database (RDB). She concluded that the student was producing an appropriate amount of talking at an average rate. The handwritten notes on Figure 18 demonstrate how the timing information, which is based on 12-minute data, is applied to the student sample, which contains 100 utterances collected in only eight minutes and 24 seconds. From the data summarized in Section II, Intelligibility, she could also see that he was about as intelligible as the average nine-year-old. The student was 91.82 percent intelligible compared to a mean of 92.35 percent.

Section III, Mazes and Overlaps, was completed next. The SLP noted that 34 of the student's utterances contained mazes, which was about one standard deviation above the mean of 25 for nine-year-olds. Therefore, further analysis of the utterances with mazes was needed and the transcript showed that
- the student used filled pauses, repetitions, and revisions (see break out on Figure 18, LSA Summary Form (completed), for counts).
- the repetitions and revisions occurred at both word and phrase levels.
- the student often started a word and then revised his word choice part of the way through production of the target word. These abandoned words were disconcerting to the listener.

When the SLP looked at all of the utterances with mazes, she found that
- there were multiple mazes in single utterances.
- pronouns were often revised.

The student interrupted the examiner frequently, as if he had to express his ideas quickly before he forgot how or what he was going to say. Ten percent of his utterances overlapped the examiner's utterances.

In Section IV of the summary form, Semantics, the SLP noted that the student's performance was similar to the mean performance of the children in the RDB. The values for Type Token Ratio; Total Words; and Different Words were all clustered about the mean. Likewise, the data from Section V, Word Lists, were in the average range.

Section VI, Syntax/Morphology, indicated the student's mean length of utterances was above the mean of 6.5 but within one standard deviation. The SLP interpreted this as average performance.

Section VII, Bound Morphemes, indicated the child used appropriate grammatical markers in all obligatory contexts except one where he omitted regular past tense (/ed). This was interpreted as an average performance.

The SLP also summarized the child's errors on the final page of the summary sheet by reviewing the transcript and listing utterances with error codes for further analysis. She categorized them as morpheme level errors (EO), word level errors (EW), pronoun errors (EP), and sentence and discourse level errors (CU and EU). She noted numerous errors at the word and discourse levels. After analyzing them carefully, she concluded that they often reflected the student's difficulty retrieving the words he needed to express his ideas.

Results of Standardized Testing

As part of the M-team assessment, several standardized tests were administered by the SLP. Results are summarized on the following page.

Test of Language Development—Primary: (Newcomer and Hammill, 1988)

Picture Vocabulary	SS	8
Oral Vocabulary	SS	9
Grammatic Understanding	SS	9
Grammatic Completion	SS	12
Sentence Imitation	SS	5
Word Discrimination	SS	10
Word Articulation	Residual, inconsistent distortion of /r/ and /l/; difficulty with multisyllabic words	

Test of Word Finding: (German, 1986)
SS 78
7 percentile
"Fast and inaccurate namer"

Peabody Picture Vocabulary Test—R: (Dunn and Dunn, 1981)
SS 104
60 percentile

Boehm Test of Basic Concepts: (Boehm, 1986)
25 percentile

WISC—R: (Wechsler, 1974)
Verbal 125
Performance 135
Full Scale 134

Academic testing confirmed teacher reports of above grade level functioning in math, and significant delays in reading (pre-primer-level performance).

M-Team

The M-team met and discussed the assessment results. The SLP presented her data from Language Sample Analysis and the standardized tests she had administered. She used the data (revisions, abandoned words, and word and discourse errors) to show how the strategies used by the student to find the words he needed interfered with communication. She and the learning disabilities specialist were able to compare observations and data which demonstrated that the student's word finding problems also resulted in reading problems: miscalling sight words, resultant inconsistent comprehension, and others. The M-team concluded that the student had a language disorder typified by word finding problems and the student was learning-disabled in reading.

Intervention Plan

Overall, the results of the language sample analysis confirmed the results of the standardized test information. The language sample, however, provided the detailed description about *how* the child's word finding problems were reflected in language use and allowed for a specific therapy program to be designed which would have the greatest chance of influencing functional communication.

The SLP targeted reducing the number of mazes, particularly revisions, as a therapy goal. The child and SLP engaged in pronoun and verb tense drill so that production of these structures became more automatic. Strategies to facilitate specific word recall were also practiced along with formulating utterances before talking, and self-monitoring overlaps and interruptions.

The process of LSA in conjunction with standardized testing also helped the child's parents better understand his communication problem. They found the use of a sample of the child's language a diagnostic tool easy to understand and valid since it reflected familiar and typical language use.

Figure 19 summarizes the steps in the LSA process in the context of a language assessment.

█ Figure 19
_____

Language Assessment Checklist

Before collecting a language sample:
- ❏ Check tape recorder, batteries, and external microphone.
- ❏ Review the noise level of the room, reduce as much as possible.
- ❏ Make sure all necessary material are available, such as paper, drawing markers, modeling clay, or story books for younger children.
- ❏ Identify the tape, noting the child's name, date of evaluation, date of birth, and sampling condition.

While recording the language sample:
- ❏ Make the child comfortable.
- ❏ Follow the sampling protocol for conversation and narrative samples as described in Section 2.
- ❏ Introduce topics as necessary to keep the interaction moving.
- ❏ Encourage spontaneous use of language. Use story books only as a last resort.

After collecting the language sample:
- ❏ Review the tape to determine if the sample is representative of the child's productive language.
- ❏ Transcribe the sample following the transcription conventions provided in Appendix C.
- ❏ Analyze the transcript by hand or using a computer-assisted strategy.
- ❏ Assemble the data into categories using the LSA Summary Form in Section 5.
- ❏ Compare the data to the Reference Database and list deficits in performance categories from LSA (for example, low MLU, low number of different words, high number of mazes).
- ❏ Summarize the standardized test results.
- ❏ Interpret the student's productive language skills relative to the language disorders taxonomy.
- ❏ Review notes from teacher(s) regarding academic and communicative performance, as well as behavior such as attention or activity level.
- ❏ Review concerns of parent(s).

❑ Synthesize the information from all assessment sources
   a. What are the child's cognitive skills compared to language skills?
   b. What is the developmental relationship between comprehension and production?
❑ Summarize recommendations to be presented at the M-team meeting regarding the child's language competency or language disorder.
❑ Participate in the M-team determination of handicapping condition(s) and need for special education intervention.
❑ If the M-team determines the child to need special education, use the specifics from LSA in developing the IEP goals, objectives, and therapy strategies.

Refer to Appendix G for additional case study data exemplifying each of the language delay and disorder types from the taxonomy presented in Section 1. These case studies will further assist the reader in applying LSA as a diagnostic strategy and will be part of training workshops that are presently being developed to facilitate interpretation of LSA.

Children Over Thirteen

Although the age ranges in the RDB do not extend above age 13, SALT analysis of language transcripts and comparisons for older students are still helpful when evaluating their language abilities. The SLP can use the Reference Database with students who are over 14, because the performances of children in the RDB seem to plateau on the majority of SALT measures, which suggests the achievement of adult competency.

Students at the secondary level have been previously identified as language disordered and thus the focus of the assessment is somewhat different. It is easier to design a probe of the student's language use when one has previous documentation of strengths and weaknesses. The M-team documents change in the student's language comprehension or production and the student's ability to apply taught strategies in communicating effectively in spite of a language disorder. Sample results are compared to previous performances.

The portions of the SALT analysis which are generally the most helpful are those tables which help to describe and quantify a disorder (maze data), those tables which help to describe the student's language complexity (conjunction data, error codes), and those tables which help to describe the student's ability to use appropriate references (pronouns, error codes). Narrative samples more closely parallel the student's use of language in academic contexts than conversation and are used more frequently at this level.

Summary

This case study (and those in Appendix G) demonstrates the power of LSA to document different types of productive language disorders and to provide the level of description necessary to develop an integrated intervention plan. In the next chapter issues concerning linguistic and cultural diversity are addressed.

References

Boehm, Ann. *Boehm Test of Basic Concepts*. San Antonio, TX: The Psychological Corporation, 1986.

Dunn, L.M. and L. Dunn. *Peabody Picture Vocabulary Test—Revised*. Circle Pines, MN: American Guidance Service, 1981.

German, D.G. *Test of Word Finding*. Allen, TX: DLM/Teaching Resources, 1986.

Newcomer, P.L. and D.D. Hammill. *Test of Language Develoment—Primary*. Second ed., Austin, TX: PRO-ED, 1988.

Wechsler, D. *Wechsler Intelligence Scale for Children—Revised*. San Antonio, TX: The Psychological Corporation, 1974.

6

Applications of LSA
for Diverse Populations

Purpose

Previous sections of this guide focused on the use of LSA in assessing children in the mainstream European-American culture. Assessing language production in diverse populations provides additional challenges which will be introduced here, although detailed coverage is beyond the scope of this document. It is critical, however, that SLPs be cautioned about the use and potential misuse of LSA, as well as the RDB, to document language deficits that may lead to the determination of an exceptional educational need (EEN).

Several groups are reviewed in this section: children who are from linguistically and culturally diverse (LCD) backgrounds; and children with cognitive disabilities, sensory disabilities; and motor disabilities. The central issues when assessing children from these groups is to distinguish these differences from language disorder.

Distinguishing Language and Cultural Differences from Language Disorders

The intent of this segment is to heighten the SLP's awareness of the relevant issues when evaluating LCD children. Failure to be sensitive to these issues could result in either an over- or under-identification of children from these groups as being language-disordered. LSA offers the opportunity to examine language performance in speaking contexts that are culturally sensitive and ensure optimal language production performance.

When considering the educational needs of children from linguistically or culturally diverse groups, it is crucial that all school staff are aware of and understand the following concepts when working with students from LCD populations. (Minnesota Department of Education, 1987)

• Lack of proficiency and skill in Standard English does not in itself make a student eligible for special education services.

• An individual who lacks Standard English skills is different from an individual with a language disorder.

• Normal sound patterns and interference from the first language in an LCD student may lead students not to discriminate Standard English sounds. This is not a learning, speech, or hearing disorder.

• It is not necessary to forget one language to learn another.

• Students may be eligible for service from both English as a Second Language (ESL) and EEN programs, having been appropriately assessed as needing both types of assistance.

• There is no such thing as a culture-free test.

• All tests given in Standard English are tests of Standard English language proficiency, regardless of the content of the test.

• Learning styles are culturally determined.

• Culturally based behavior may mislead teaching staff to believe an LCD student has an EEN.

• The culture of an American school may not be compatible with an LCD student's culturally based learning styles.

• One cannot assume that parents of culturally and/or linguistically different students have the same perception or attitude toward schools as parents of the mainstream culture.

- The parents and family members of an LCD student have valuable information which is essential in planning an appropriate educational plan for that student.

Schools have a responsibility to serve students in the least restrictive environment. Therefore, school personnel should make every effort to gather all relevant data on the student. School staff must be prepared to modify and adapt the regular education setting and curriculum. When appropriate, the school must develop an ESL program. Only after exploring these various routes can the school appropriately consider an EEN.

The primary problems faced by educators when evaluating the language performance of LCD populations are a general lack of understanding about the differences among cultural groups, lack of understanding the process of learning English as a second language, and a lack of specific diagnostic tools to help distinguish those students having difficulty learning English from those who are having difficulty learning *any* language. Cultural and linguistic diversity significantly affects language learning and performance in school. (Fradd and Weismantel, 1989; Garcia and Flores, 1986; Hamayan and Damico, 1991) LSA can assist in identifying children with potential EEN from those whose language skills are culturally or linguistically different. A task force of Minnesota educators reported:

While it is important to understand basic cultural differences that an LCD student may exhibit, it is equally important to recognize the individuality of each LCD student and to avoid inaccurate, stereotypical expectations. Each LCD student may be at a different stage of adjustment to U.S. schools and customs. The age at which students have experienced certain cultural and personal events may affect their present reactions. It is inappropriate to expect all students from a similar language and cultural background to demonstrate similar characteristics and behaviors. ("All LCD students do well in math," or "All the LCD students are shy and well-behaved.")

Language is an important aspect of culture. Culturally different students may also be linguistically different students. LCD students, as determined above, will naturally have difficulty in an academic setting if they are unable to communicate in Standard English in the four basic skill areas of listening, speaking, reading, and writing. Instruction in Standard English will require that all four areas be very well developed before an LCD student is able to successfully perform in an English academic setting. Often, difficulties that are common in the process of acquiring a new language are often mistaken for learning, hearing, or speech disabilities, which they are not. It is therefore essential that LCD students be assessed in their first language and that basic information regarding a second language acquisition be understood by all of those observing and assessing the student. (Minnesota Department of Education, 1987)

The process of determining whether a student has an EEN involves several steps
- Pre-referral (adaptations and modifications)
- Referral
- Assessment
- M-team eligibility determination
- IEP development
- Placement

The assessment and identification process for students with limited English proficiency is seen as being even more difficult than it is for English proficient students. This occurs because of the added cultural and first language influence that SLPs must distinguish from the student's opportunity and ability to learn English.

A beginning step in the overall procedure is the completion of a case history focusing on the student's primary culture and language, including developmental milestones; general health; medical background; family history; previous educational experience; as well as current English language proficiency of the family. The case history should recognize and encompass important cultural information, standards, attitudes, child-rearing practices, and beliefs and values that affect language development. (Prutting, 1983; Mattes and Omark, 1984; Iglesias, 1985) Collectively, these variables shape and define rules of social interaction and language use which influence child performance during the assessment process and in the classroom. (Walker, 1985; Mattes and Omark, 1984; Erickson-Good, 1985; Hamayan and Damico, 1991)

Community leaders, parents (through interpreters when necessary), ESL teachers, and classroom teachers are resources available to SLPs who can offer insight into the role of culture on the individual student's language and school success. Increased awareness of these factors enhances sensitivity in the selection of appropriate topics and materials to aid the evaluation process and interpretation of results. (Hamayan and Damico, 1991)

It is important to compile a comprehensive language profile of abilities that includes phonology, syntax, semantics at the lexical and sentential levels, and the social use of language in both comprehension and production. Non-verbal cognitive status combined with the child's overall ability also needs to be included in the profile.

Using an Interpreter

When the SLP is neither fluent in the student's primary language or familiar with the student's culture, it is critical that a qualified interpreter be used in the evaluation. Ideally, interpreters are adults who have little or no prior knowledge of the student. Relatives or friends may be too accustomed to the child to base their interpretations on language alone, or they may be unwilling to indicate deficiencies in their own family.

Sensitivity to gender, age, and religious and political beliefs, as well as social or tribal status are also important. The school district should make a culturally appropriate choice of interpreter. Socio-status and life experiences play a role in determining cultural appropriateness. As in all societies, there are arbitrary reasons for associating or disassociating with different groups of people. Although the particular reasons may seem unfair or confusing, school districts must respect the sensitivities of the family and work with a mutually acceptable choice of interpreter. The initial meeting between the SLP and the interpreter is an excellent time to plan methods of elicitation and response.

When interpreters are not professionals with the skills, knowledge, and training in educational assessment, it is necessary for the SLP to clearly define the purpose of assessment and explain, to some degree, both the theory and practice involved. If necessary, some fundamental explanation of the philosophy of EEN should be offered during this training.

Interpreters should know why they are gathering information and how they should elicit responses that will be useful. Both exact translations of the student's language and general impressions on the part of the interpreter are valuable: the SLP should help the interpreter know when each form of information is appropriate. Interpreters should be prepared to offer an opinion on whether the student is having problems because of a disability or simply because of a bi-cultural life experience which often loses pieces of each culture in the mix.

Parents

Although LCD parents are not appropriate interpreters they maintain the same role that every parent in Wisconsin holds when educational decisions must be made for their children. Their sometimes limited knowledge of culture and education practices in the United States makes it imperative for the SLP to strive to communicate with them as fully as possible. School staff must take the time and feel the responsibility to educate LCD parents about both the programs offered to their children, and their right to accept or decline these services.

Using LSA to Identify and Describe Disordered Language Performance

There are few standardized, norm-referenced, speech and language measurement tools designed specifically for LCD students. Content and norms of standardized assessment tools typically will not account for the possible differences in structure, meaning, and social use of language or the prosodic characteristics unique to LCD children. These tools will not offer insight into either the student's range of linguistic performance for both the primary and secondary language, and will under-represent the student's capacity for language learning.

Given the restrictions of standardized assessment tools used in the evaluation of language for an LCD student, more direct quantitative measures of performance such as language sampling have been endorsed by a number of authorities in the field. (Mattes and Omark, 1984; Langdon, 1983; Leonard and Weiss, 1983; Gallagher, 1983; Fey, 1986; Hamayan and Damico, 1991) Use of these tools allows for assessment of language in both the primary or first language (L1) and the second language (L2) regardless of linguistic dominance or proficiency. (Hamayan and Damico, 1991)

Use of language sampling in both the first language (L1) and its various dialects and second language (L2) allows the child to demonstrate the true range of language abilities required for communicating a variety of messages essential for school progress. (Naremore, 1985; Van Kleeck and Richardson, 1989) In addition, language sampling can be used to document linguistic change over time serving as indicators of the student's language growth and development relative to school performance. (Wallach and Miller, 1988)

Performance on language samples in L1, other dialects, and L2 can offer comprehensive information about how the child incorporates all language domains into effective communication. (Prutting, 1983; Erickson-Good, 1985; Oller, 1983; Grosjean, 1989) Students who exhibit difficulties in language and communication development in both languages are more easily identified when data on the student's performance is available in both languages. Performance deficits in Standard English, when it is the second language, may be associated with second language acquisition rather than deviant language performance. Every student will present a unique assessment and interpretation problem: frequently the results are not clear-cut. The use of LSA will improve the level of specificity of the data available for interpretation. In many cases the identification of disordered language performance is significantly improved because of the use of LSA procedures. (Miller, 1991; Lund and Duchan, 1988; Leonard and Weiss, 1983)

See Appendix D, Resources, for Owen's summaries of specific dialectic differences among Standard Black English, Hispanic English, and Asian-American English. Owen's material does not include information on American Indian language.

It is surprising to find how little specific and directly applicable information exists on the dialectical or language differences of American Indian children by tribe or band, or the problems they encounter learning Standard English as a second language. Research found studies that referenced Navaho and Ute but nothing that gave lexicons of Wisconsin tribes or bands. Because of the great number and varieties of American Indian languages and dialectical variations of Standard English—"Indian English"—the question itself may be no different than asking what problems would anyone face who is learning English as a second language. The Wisconsin Department of Public Instruction has developed publications that offer information on American Indian culture in Wisconsin, yet their objectives do not cover an in-depth linguistic study of any specific clan, band, or tribe.

Wisconsin school districts are currently participating in a grant project which seeks to create language sampling methods and conditions which are culturally sensitive. The DPI hopes that the information derived by sampling a large number of American Indian, African-American, Hispanic, and Asian-American students will provide a range of diagnostically helpful information. Obviously, the degree of assimilation to the mainstream culture and language that the child and the family have undergone will have a significant effect on the child's language development and production. American Indian English, African-American English, Hispanic English, and Asian-American English are genuine phenomena, best received as non-standard, but not as sub-standard English or disordered performance.

Evaluating Students with Cognitive, Sensory, and Motor Disabilities

Cognitive Disabilities

SLPs must exercise caution when using the RDB to interpret the performance of students with cognitive disabilities. Interpretation of the language performance of these students can be compared to either chronological or mental age. The mental age (MA) performance rather than the chronological age (CA) is the preferred metric of comparison with the RDB because the rate of language development has greater correlation to cognitive skills than to chronological skills. The Reference Database does not include data on mental age; it is organized only by chronological age (CA). While it is not unreasonable to use its CA-based charts, as a cautious first step, to interpret the language performance of a student with a cognitive disability, the SLP must assume that the CA is commensurate with the MA in typically developing students. When the child is identified as cognitively disabled, the SLP should use the child's MA area of strength (non-verbal or verbal) and compare it with the same CA of a typically developing child. For example, a child who has a chronological age of ten years and a mental age of seven years should be assessed using data from the group of seven-year-olds.

Sensory Disabilities

A student who is deaf or hard-of-hearing (DHH) communicates using spoken language requires an assessment that is similar to the assessment of a student with normal hearing. Useful information regarding the expressive spoken English abilities of the student who is DHH can be gained by completing LSA and by comparing his or her spoken language sample to those of other students in the RDB.

As with any student who exhibits deficits in speech production, special consideration must be given to how the ability of the child who is DHH to produce the sounds of the language affects the outcome of the language analysis. First, in a given sample, unless at least 70 to 80 percent of the utterances are intelligible, the validity of the subsequent analysis is highly questionable.

A second consideration regarding the speech production of a student who is DHH is its effect on the student's ability to produce the various function words and morphological markers of English. For example, if the child produces "a" for "the," a determination must be made as to whether this is a speech production error (like an inability or inconsistent ability to produce the "the" phoneme) or a language error. Similarly, if the student evidences errors on third person present conjugation and/or regular pluralization, this may be the result of an articulation error (such as difficulty producing the "s" and/or "z" phonemes) rather than a language deficit per se.

When analyzing the language of students who are DHH who use sign language, the SLP must determine where the child's language falls on the continuum from English to American Sign Language (a language with its own set of syntactic and morphologic rules which are distinct from English) because LSA must be performed relative to the language system the child uses. Because the RDB contains information about English only, it would be inappropriate to relate it to a student who uses American Sign Language (ASL). Only in cases where a student is exposed to and expected to use a strict form of manually coded English, signing all of the lexical, syntactic, and morphologic aspects of English, would it be appropriate to use the RDB for comparative purposes. For the many students who are DHH who communicate using features of both ASL and English, it would be useful to analyze their abilities in both of these languages.

Often it is helpful to video-, as well as audio-tape the student, because watching the child speak often facilitates the transcriber's ability to understand the child. The transcription and analysis of sign language samples naturally requires videotaping of the student and is a time-consuming and nonstandardized procedure. When attempting transcription and analysis of these samples, a number of important issues must be considered. First, the transcriber must be fluent in the sign language or system used by the student. Second, when dealing with samples of ASL, analysis and interpretation are often difficult and somewhat subjective because normative data regarding the developmental acquisition of ASL is sparse. In addition, there is a very limited pool of individuals who are qualified to undertake such an analysis because it requires thorough knowledge of the linguistic structure and features of ASL. Many other issues, beyond the scope of this manual, must be considered when transcribing and analyzing sign language.

Students who are blind or visually impaired require an assessment that is similar to their fully sighted peers, but the SLP must keep in mind that language acquisition may be different for blind children. One can assume that just as vision influences cognitive development, it also influences the strategies children use in acquiring and using language. As in the case of students who are DHH, LSA is extremely useful in the assessment of students who are blind and visually impaired, as long as the SLP is sensitive to the students' visual limitations. The Wisconsin Department of Public Instruction's *A Guide to Curriculum Planning for Visually Impaired Students* offers the following suggestions.

Familiarizing oneself with the background information concerning the visual diagnosis and consulting with the services of the teacher of the visually impaired will assist in determining the adaptations needed during the assessment process . . . . The following are linguistic strategies which may be characteristics of some blind children:

• frequently observed is "verbalism," a parrot-like repetition of words without understanding or meaning.

• both immediate and delayed echolalia are frequently observed in visually impaired children.

• blind children use descriptive color words less frequently than do their sighted peers; however, establishing color concepts needs to be addressed on an individual basis.

- blind children use fewer "see" verbs than do sighted children and many of the "see" verbs appear in grammatical constructions with meanings unlike the traditional meaning used by sighted peers.
- blind children are more prone to personal reference mistakes but demonstrate potential for proficiency in this area.
- blind children may use more question forms to secure information, for orientation purposes, and for conventional control and maintenance.
- blind children may use fewer question forms due to cognitive development or lack of experience.
- blind children make minimal use of communicative gestures with or without verbalization. This can result in unresolved confusion of word meaning. (Tapp, Wilhelm, and Loveless, 1991)

These differences are seen in oral language production and would be documented through the use of LSA. The language sample analysis should be coupled with an evaluation of non-verbal, gesture, and pragmatic skills. LSA is a valuable assessment tool assuming the SLP remains sensitive to the impact of the student's visual acuity and exercises caution when comparing standard results to the RDB.

Motor Disabilities

Children with motor problems are of concern where disabilities may affect the speech motor system, limiting the nature and amount of productive language and reducing speech intelligibility. Lack of intelligibility of speech limits the SLP's ability to perform LSA, because it affects judgments of word, phrase, and clausal segments. Again, intelligibility that is less than 70 to 80 percent precludes analysis of productive language. The diagnostic problem is the differentiation between deficits in productive language that are linguistic and representational in origin, and those that are a result of a motor control deficit.

Summary

This section has briefly outlined the major diagnostic concerns that SLPs associate using LSA with students whose additional disabilities and cultural differences influence their performance. These data can be very useful for interpretation of a child's language production as long as SLPs understand the conditional nature of the interpretation and exercise the proper caution. In summary, the following steps are recommended when evaluating LCD students:
- Review all assessment data relative to the student's culture to assist in interpretation of disordered performance and EEN.
- Compare L1, or its dialect, and L2 to note consistency of error patterns.
- Assess both conversation and narration to provide opportunity for optimal language use.
- Contrast conversational and narrative performance using language and communication profile.
- Use the RDB only as a guideline for performance, because these data are a product of mainstream culture sampling conditions and subjects.

The identification and use of appropriate LSA methods and procedures for distinguishing language difference from language disorder in culturally diverse populations continues to be a priority in Wisconsin. The Department of Public Instruction is currently funding a multi-year grant project that explores these issues.

Figure 20

Sample Checklist of Information Needed*

Name _____

Student Number _____

There is documentation that:

❑ The student has been assessed by ESL or bilingual education staff and determined to currently be linguistically and culturally diverse (LCD).

❑ The student was born in another country, had a first language other than English or has a cultural background very different from school peers, suggesting that nondiscriminatory assessment procedures would be appropriate.

❑ First language proficiency has been determined.

❑ Oral English proficiency has been assessed and recorded in the areas of (1) comprehension, (2) pronunciation, (3) syntax, (4) vocabulary, and (5) pragmatics.

❑ The best language of instruction for basic skills and content areas has been documented.

❑ The student has had opportunity to learn by being provided content area instruction appropriate to his/her English proficiency and academic performance level.

❑ Appropriate ESL and/or bilingual education services have been provided.

❑ Appropriate adaptations and modifications have been carried out.

There is documentation that all special education assessments were accomplished in a nondiscriminatory manner:

❑ Assessments were completed in the native language when appropriate.

❑ Assistance of native language interpreters or cultural representatives was provided when appropriate.

❑ Comprehension of basic academic concepts in the native language and in English has been determined.

❑ A variety of assessment procedures were used.

❑ Results of formal academic assessments have been reported in terms of curriculum or criterion-referenced measures rather than norm-referenced scores.

❑ Results of formal intellectual assessments have been reported as an estimated range of ability rather than as norm-referenced scores.

❑ Information from student's family and home community environment has been obtained as part of the assessment.

❑ Information regarding the student's health, developmental and educational history has been considered.

There is documentation that procedural safeguards were followed:

❑ General education and ESL or bilingual education staff were on the M-team.

❑ Due process forms were provided to parents or guardians in the native language in written translation or oral interpretation as appropriate.

❑ Communications (e.g., phone, in-person) and meetings with the student and/or parents included native language interpretation when needed.

❑ All relevant areas of assessment have been conducted as suggested by state criteria.

❑ Eligibility decisions were made by the team based upon multiple assessments including formal and informal measures, and upon information provided by the parents.

---

* *Service Delivery Guidelines for LEP Students with Special Education Needs*. St. Paul, MN: Minnesota Department of Education. ©1987, pp. 50-51. Reprinted with permission.

References

Erickson-Good, J. "How Many Languages Do You Speak? An Overview of Bilingual Education." *Topics in Language Disorders* 5 (1985), pp. 1-14.

Fey, M. *Language Intervention with Young Children*. San Diego, CA: College Hill Press, 1986.

Fletcher, J. D. *What Problems Do American Indians Have with English?* Orem, UT: WICAT, Inc., 1983.

Fradd, S. and M. J. Weismantel. *Meeting the Needs of Culturally and Linguistically Different Students: A Handbook for Educators*. San Diego, CA: Singular Publishing Group, 1989.

Garcia, E. and B. Flores, eds. *Language and Literacy Research in Bilingual Education*. Tempe, AZ: Arizona State University Center for Bilingual Education, 1986.

Gallagher, T. "Pre-Assessment: A Procedure for Accommodating Language Use Variability." In *Pragmatic Assessment and Intervention: Issues in Language*. Eds. T. Gallagher and C. Prutting. San Diego, CA: College Hill Press, 1983, pp. 1-28.

Grosjean, F. "Neurolinguists, Beware! The Bilingual Is Not Two Monolinguals In One Person." *Brain and Language* 36 (1989), pp. 3-15.

Hamayan, E. and J. Damico. *Limiting Bias in the Assessment of Bilingual Students*. San Diego, CA: Singular Publishing Group, Inc., 1991.

Iglesias, A. "Communication in the Home and Classroom: Match or Mismatch?" *Topics in Language Disorders* 5 (1985), pp. 29-41.

Langdon, H. "Assessment and Intervention Strategies for the Bilingual Language Disordered Student." *Exceptional Children* 50 (1983), pp. 37-46.

Leonard, L. and A. Weiss. "Application of Nonstandardized Assessment Procedures to Diverse Linguistic Populations." *Topics in Language Disorders* 3 (1983), pp. 35-45.

Lund, N. and J. Duchan. *Assessing Children's Language in Naturalistic Contexts*. Englewood Cliffs, NJ: Prentice-Hall, 1988.

Mattes, L. and D. Omark. *Speech and Language Assessment for the Bilingual Handicapped*. San Diego, CA: College Hill Press, 1984.

Miller, J. "Quantifying Productive Language Disorder." In *Research on Child Language Disorders: A Decade of Progress*. Ed. J. Miller. Austin, TX: PRO-ED, 1991, pp. 211-220.

Naremore, R. "Explorations of Language Use: Pragmatic Mapping in L1 and L2." *Topics in Language Disorders* 5 (1985), pp. 66-79.

Oller, J. "Testing Proficiencies and Diagnosing Language Disorders in Bilingual Children." In *The Bilingual Exceptional Child*. Eds. D. Omark and J. Erickson-Good. San Diego, CA: College Hill Press, 1983, pp. 69-88.

Prutting, C. "Assessing Communicative Behavior Using a Language Sample." In *The Bilingual Exceptional Child*. Eds. D. Omark and J. Erickson-Good. San Diego, CA: College Hill Press, 1983, pp. 89-99.

A Resource Handbook for the Assessment and Identification of LEP students with Special Education Needs. St. Paul, MN: Minnesota Department of Education, 1987.

Tapp, Kenneth L., James G. Wilhelm, and Lori J. Loveless. *A Guide to Curriculum Planning for Visually Impaired Students*. Madison, WI: Wisconsin Department of Public Instruction, 1991, pp. 146-148.

Van Kleeck, A. and A. Richardson. "Developmental Assessment of Speech and Language." In *Developmental Assessment in Clinical Child Psychology*. Eds. J. Johnson and J. Goldman. New York: Permagon Press, 1989, pp. 186-210.

Walker, C. "Learning English: The Southeast Asian Refugee Experience." *Topics in Language Disorders* 5 (1985), pp. 53-65.

Wallach, G. and L. Miller. *Language Intervention and Academic Success*. San Diego, CA: Singular Publishing Group, Inc., 1988.

7

LSA and the M-Team Process

Determining Exceptional Educational Need
Increasing the Consistency of Identification
Final Remarks

Determining Exceptional Educational Need

The Wisconsin rules and regulations that implement exceptional education law specify a school district's responsibility to provide a free, appropriate public education for all children and youth who have been evaluated and identified as having a disability and an exceptional educational need (EEN). These rules further specify the minimum criteria for the determination of a handicapping condition and eligibility for exceptional education in the area of speech and language. The identified child must exhibit a significant "delay or deviance in the acquisition of prelinguistic skills, receptive skills, or expressive skills or both of oral communication." (PI 11.35(2)(e)1) *Children are not served in special education when they have only a mild speech and language problem.* Speech and language programs are provided by districts to students whose oral communication disorders significantly interfere with their ability to succeed in their educational setting and so require exceptional education.

A comprehensive evaluation, consisting of formal and informal assessments of the child's oral communication abilities as they relate to peer and adult interactions and the child's ability to function as a learner in his or her present educational program, must provide the information through which an M-team determines a handicapping condition and a need for special education.

LSA will assist the SLP in obtaining substantive data which more clearly addresses the determination of a handicapping condition. The information which describes how a speech and language disorder interferes with the ability to handle language demands across environments, something which test scores alone cannot provide, is critical to this decision. The Reference Database contained in Appendix A provides the information needed to document a significant discrepancy between a child's language production skills from those of typically developing children of the same age. The RDB's use across the state of Wisconsin can help increase the consistency of identifying students with language disabilities by focusing diagnostic efforts on the language used in functional contexts and comparing it to a representative sample of typically developing children in the state.

While determining eligibility and the need for special education, it is critical that the SLP consider more than the degree or severity of the language deviation. The process must also consider the degree to which the speech or language deviation interferes with the child's ability to acquire and utilize knowledge, maintain satisfactory social relationships, or have sound emotional development. (Refer to Figure 21 for relevant indicators.)

Figure 21

Indicators for Determining a Handicapping Condition

A. Does the communication disorder interfere with peer and adult interactions in school, home, and community?   YES / NO

    1. Parents have voiced their concern about their child's communication problem and its effect on them and/or other family members.
Explain: (cite observable/measurable events)

    2. Teachers have voiced their concern about the child's communication problem and its effect on them and/or classmates.
Explain:

    3. This student has experienced negative peer group reaction or ridicule during speaking situations or because of his/her communication problem.
Explain:

    4. This student is aware of his/her communication problem and is concerned about it.
Explain:

    5. This student uses a lot of gestures instead of speech to communicate.
Explain:

B. Does the communication disorder interfere with the student's ability to function as a learner in his/her present educational program or setting?   YES / NO

    1. This student's communication problems interferes with intelligibility or makes it difficult to understand the content of his/her verbal message.
Explain: (cite observable/measurable events)

    2. Does this student avoid speaking in class?
Explain:

    3. Does this student exhibit observable frustration or anxiety when speaking or attempting to speak?
Explain:

4. Is this student's communication problem more pronounced during any particular time of the day?
Explain:

5. Is this student usually able to follow your oral directions?
Explain:

6. The student's communication problem occurs within educational areas such as spelling, concept work, reading, listening skills, math concepts, etc.
Explain:

7. This student's reading and/or spelling skills reflect his or her articulation errors.
Explain:

8. Does this student appear to focus on only part of what is said, and therefore sometimes misinterprets information?
Explain:

9. During class discussions is the student able to contribute to the topic being discussed?
Explain:

10. Is the student able to respond appropriately to questions asked?
Explain:

11. Is the student able to express ideas and experiences in a logical and sequential fashion with clarity and accuracy?
Explain:

12. Is the student able to get information or assistance by asking appropriate questions?
Explain:

13. Does the student use grammatically intact sentences and sentence fragments which are appropriate to the context?
Explain:

14. Are there any other observations relating to the communication skills of the student which should be noted?

Although some SLPs may *wish* for a specific standard deviation cut off or some "magic number" which would indicate the level at which a child becomes disabled and requires special education, this is not always in the best interests of the individual child. **All** districts must serve **only** children identified as disabled in oral communication and needing exceptional education.

The following figure provides a visual representation of the referral through placement process as defined in Wisconsin Administrative Code PI 11. The points below are necessary considerations during the Referral through Placement Process (in Figure 22).

- Does the student meet established minimum criteria for determination of handicapping condition and eligibility for special education?
- How or in what way is the communication disorder handicapping to the student?
- Does the student's communication disorder necessitate specially designed instruction or can the student's communication disorder be handled by others responsible for his or her present instructional program?
- How would essential elements (instructional elements of a proposed speech and language program) differ from what is or could be provided to the student in his or her present educational placement or setting?
- Exceptional Educational Need (EEN) programming.
- Non-EEN Recommendations

PI 1104.(5)(b)1-3

(b) If an M-team finds that a child is not a child with EEN the M-team report shall also include the following:

1. An identification of the child's non-exceptional education needs.

2. A referral to any programs, other than special education programs, offered by the board from which the child may benefit.

3. Information about any programs and services other than those offered by the board that the M-team is aware of that may provide a benefit to the child.

Referral through Placement Process

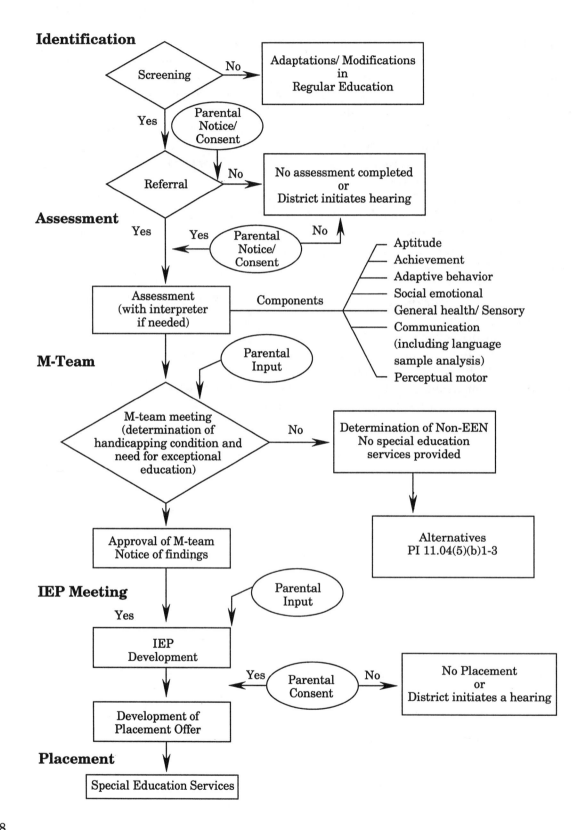

Increasing the Consistency of Identification

Inconsistent or inappropriate identification of children as having a speech and language handicapping condition is extremely costly in terms of professional and fiscal resources. The delivery of inappropriate or unnecessary intervention is also costly. The detailed description of language performance that LSA provides helps to address appropriate, consistent identification and development of intervention plans.

During therapy, the data obtained from LSA provides a reference point for monitoring progress, revising goals, or dismissing the child from the program. LSA provides a tangible description of the student's progress and is directly applicable to the annual IEP review.

SLPs are aware of both the fiscal and human costs of inappropriate identification. They witness the frustration of students who continue to have increasing difficulties throughout their school years, sometimes leading to a need for other remedial or EEN programs, because their language and communication problems were not accurately identified and addressed. Practicing SLPs who routinely use LSA are also discovering that some children who, by standardized test scores alone, would otherwise have been identified as EEN do not need placement in a speech and language program when a detailed analysis of their language has been provided. When LSA is applied, it can directly document both the disability or the lack of a disability. These are the real benefits of language sample analysis.

Final Remarks

Language Sample Analysis (LSA) as presented in this guide has been used in the Madison Metropolitan School District (on a district-wide basis) for the last five years and in CESA 9 for one year.

It has been used consistently by a very diverse group of SLPs including some who are very experienced (over 20 years in the field) and by SLPs in their first job position.

As a finale to this guide, the LSA Task Force would like to share some thoughts and feelings that these "pioneers" in the Wisconsin LSA process have expressed as an encouragement to each reader—to persevere in learning about and using these LSA methodologies.

LSA looks at the child's whole language system—how he [or she] puts it all together. It's much more valid than tests which ask the child to focus on one aspect of language at a time, and respond using single words or phrases.

> Rebecca Zutter-Brose, Huegel Elementary School
> Madison Metropolitan School District

LSA has made me a better pathologist because I've learned a lot more about oral language development. SALT has freed my time to do the interpretation instead of just counting words.

> Dee Boyd, Sherman Middle School
> Madison Metropolitan School District

I love being able to let my students pick what topics they want to talk about. Most standardized tests are totally teacher directed. Language samples allow the children to share what is important or interesting to them. I get to know the children as well as learn about their language skills.

Lynda Ruchti, Kennedy Elementary School
Madison Metropolitan School District

One of the most important features (of language sample analysis) may be that it is a language measuring tool that is parent-friendly because it does not require special knowledge to understand it.

Marianne Reeves, East High School
Madison Metropolitan School District

This has been the most fascinating diagnostic tool I've ever used . . . . I'm learning so much. CESA 9's utilization of LSA and the transcription lab is moving us to new levels of consistency in assessment.

Kathy Bertolino, CESA 9

It is the wish of the LSA Task Force that the use of this guide and following training will bring each of you similar positive feelings!

8

Appendixes

Reference Database*

Subjects

Subjects were 266 children from Madison Wisconsin and CESA 9 three to 13 years of age. All children were drawn from preschools in Madison or the Madison metropolitan public school system or CESA 9. Subjects were sampled from the diverse socio-economic areas represented in these areas. The subject population is a random sample reflecting the diverse socio-economic status of Wisconsin.

Age Group	Mean Age	Age Range	Male	Female	Total
3-year-olds	3.1	2.7 - 3.4	22	20	42
4-year-olds	4.0	3.7 - 4.3	18	12	30
5-year-olds	5.4	5.2 - 5.5	15	13	28
6-year olds	5.9	5.5 - 6.4	17	18	35
7-year-olds	7.1	6.7 - 7.5	12	30	35
9-year-olds	9.1	8.8 - 9.4	20	17	50
11-year-olds	11.1	10.8 - 11.3	14	13	27
13-year-olds	13.0	12.8 - 13.2	14	13	27

Terminology

In the Reference Database, the statistical abbreviations that run horizontally across the Content-Rate Summaries are the following: Mean, SD, SD–, SD+, %SD, R–, R+. "Mean" refers to the average number for each variable. "SD" is an abbreviation for the standard deviation from the mean. "SD–" provides the reader with the figure that is one standard deviation below the mean, while "SD+" shows the figure that is one standard deviation above the mean. "%SD" refers to subject variability; when the percentage is low, the database judgments are more reliable. "R–" refers to the lowest performance for that age group, and "R+" refers to the highest performance of the age group.

---

* Jon F. Miller. *Salt Reference Database Project*, Language Analysis Laboratory, Waisman Center on Mental Retardation and Human Development, University of Wisconsin. Madison, WI, 1992. Reprinted with permission.

Content and Rate Summary / 3-Year-Olds

(Conversation N=42)

Variables	Content 100 Utterance Samples						
	Mean	SD	SD–	SD+	%SD	R–	R+
Mean Length of Utterance (MLU)	3.38	0.59	2.78	3.97	18%	2	5
Type Token Ratio	0.48	0.05	0.43	0.54	11%	0	1
Total Words	310	54	256	365	17%	222	443
Different Words	118	20	98	139	17%	75	178
Utterances with Mazes	16	7	8	23	47%	0	33
Utterances with Overlaps	10	4	6	15	42%	2	20

Bound Morphemes Frequency

Regular Past	2	2	0	3	122%	0	8
Plural	7	4	3	11	53%	0	17
Possessive	1	2	-1	3	177%	0	9
Third Person Singular	2	3	0	5	121%	0	13
Present Progressive	3	2	1	5	71%	0	8

Utterance Content

Personal Pronouns (Total)	44	14	30	58	32%	15	73
(Types)	7	2	6	9	24%	4	11
Total Questions	11	8	3	20	75%	0	40
(WH Total)	7	6	1	13	87%	0	25
(WH Types)	2	1	1	4	61%	0	5
Negatives (Total)	12	6	6	18	52%	1	25
(Types)	4	2	3	6	38%	1	7
Conjunctions (Total)	12	7	5	19	59%	1	24
(Types)	3	1	2	5	47%	1	6
Modals (Total)	4	4	0	8	95%	0	15
(Types)	1	1	1	2	62%	0	3

Variables	Rate 12 Minute Samples						
	Mean	SD	SD–	SD+	%SD	R–	R+
Total Utterances	137	34	102	171	25%	55	216
Complete and Intelligible Utterances	120	30	90	151	25%	46	176
Total Words	374	110	265	484	29%	110	600
Different Words	132	31	101	163	23%	59	209
Mean Length of Utterance (MLU)	3.40	0.62	2.78	4.02	18%	3	5
Between Utterance Pauses	35.55	17.91	17.64	53.46	50%	3	82
Between Utterance Pause Time	2.25	1.31	0.94	3.57	58%	0.1	5.2
Within Utterance Pauses	1.12	1.85	-0.73	2.97	165%	0	7
Within Utterance Pause Time	0.05	0.09	-0.04	0.14	174%	0.0	0.3
Words per Minute	38.47	11.53	26.95	50.00	30%	10	63
Utterances per Minute	11.38	2.85	8.53	14.23	25%	5	18

Content and Rate Summary / 4-Year-Olds

(Conversation N=30)

Variables	Content 100 Utterance Samples						
	Mean	SD	SD–	SD+	%SD	R–	R+
Mean Length of Utterance (MLU)	4.22	1.02	3.20	5.23	24%	3	7
Type Token Ratio	0.48	0.06	0.42	0.54	12%	0	1
Total Words	384	90	295	474	23%	234	624
Different Words	144	26	117	170	18%	99	217
Utterances with Mazes	19	10	9	29	52%	6	49
Utterances with Overlaps	14	6	8	20	43%	6	33
Bound Morphemes Frequency							
Regular Past	2	2	0	3	110%	0	6
Plural	11	7	4	18	62%	2	32
Possessive	1	1	0	2	148%	0	5
Third Person Singular	4	3	1	7	77%	0	11
Present Progressive	3	3	0	6	90%	0	12
Utterance Content							
Personal Pronouns (Total)	57	17	40	74	30%	27	91
(Types)	8	2	7	10	21%	4	11
Total Questions	6	5	2	11	72%	0	21
(WH Total)	4	3	1	6	73%	0	10
(WH Types)	2	1	1	3	57%	0	4
Negatives (Total)	14	6	8	19	41%	4	26
(Types)	5	2	3	6	36%	2	8
Conjunctions (Total)	24	17	7	41	72%	6	74
(Types)	4	1	3	6	28%	2	7
Modals (Total)	4	3	1	7	74%	0	11
(Types)	2	1	1	3	58%	0	4

Variables	Rate 12 Minute Samples						
	Mean	SD	SD–	SD+	%SD	R–	R+
Total Utterances	138	33	104	171	24%	74	215
Complete and Intelligible Utterances	127	33	94	160	26%	63	199
Total Words	476	129	347	606	27%	186	749
Different Words	163	31	132	195	19%	84	254
Mean Length of Utterance (MLU)	4.20	0.98	3.23	5.18	23%	3	7
Between Utterance Pauses	25.63	13.40	12.23	39.03	52%	5	58
Between Utterance Pause Time	1.74	1.16	0.58	2.89	67%	0.2	4.6
Within Utterance Pauses	0.83	1.05	-0.22	1.89	126%	0	4
Within Utterance Pause Time	0.05	0.07	-0.03	0.12	158%	0.0	0.3
Words per Minute	47.23	12.08	35.15	59.32	26%	17	69
Utterances per Minute	11.48	2.79	8.69	14.27	24%	6	18

Content and Rate Summary / 5-Year-Olds

(Conversation N=28)

Variables	Content 100 Utterance Samples						
	Mean	SD	SD–	SD+	%SD	R–	R+
Mean Length of Utterance (MLU)	5.71	0.91	4.81	6.62	16%	4	7
Type Token Ratio	0.45	0.05	0.40	0.50	11%	0	1
Total Words	520	81	439	602	16%	380	645
Different Words	181	25	156	206	14%	117	228
Utterances with Mazes	22	9	13	31	42%	7	40
Utterances with Overlaps	11	6	6	17	49%	0	22
Bound Morphemes Frequency							
Regular Past	4	3	1	6	75%	0	10
Plural	15	8	7	22	51%	2	31
Possessive	2	2	0	5	102%	0	9
Third Person Singular	7	5	2	11	73%	1	23
Present Progressive	5	4	1	8	73%	0	16
Utterance Content							
Personal Pronouns (Total)	81	15	67	96	18%	55	110
(Types)	10	1	8	11	15%	6	12
Total Questions	7	6	1	13	81%	0	22
(WH Total)	4	4	0	8	89%	0	15
(WH Types)	2	1	1	3	56%	0	4
Negatives (Total)	13	5	7	18	41%	4	23
(Types)	5	1	4	7	27%	3	8
Conjunctions (Total)	42	18	24	60	43%	11	76
(Types)	7	1	5	8	20%	4	10
Modals (Total)	6	4	2	10	72%	0	14
(Types)	2	1	1	4	51%	0	5

Variables	Rate 12 Minute Samples						
	Mean	SD	SD–	SD+	%SD	R–	R+
Total Utterances	149	27	123	176	18%	108	211
Complete and Intelligible Utterances	139	27	112	166	19%	99	193
Total Words	724	187	537	911	26%	423	1140
Different Words	219	39	179	258	18%	144	315
Mean Length of Utterance (MLU)	5.71	0.87	4.84	6.58	15%	4	7
Between Utterance Pauses	21.61	12.54	9.07	34.15	58%	4	49
Between Utterance Pause Time	1.26	0.86	0.40	2.12	68%	0.2	3.6
Within Utterance Pauses	2.43	2.96	-0.53	5.39	122%	0	10
Within Utterance Pause Time	0.15	0.21	-0.05	0.36	135%	0.0	0.7
Words per Minute	69.48	17.69	51.79	87.18	25%	40	105
Utterances per Minute	12.48	2.24	10.23	14.72	18%	9	18

Content and Rate Summary / 6-Year-Olds

(Conversation N=35)

Variables	Content 100 Utterance Samples						
	Mean	**SD**	**SD–**	**SD+**	**%SD**	**R–**	**R+**
Mean Length of Utterance (MLU)	5.49	0.97	4.52	6.46	18%	3	8
Type Token Ratio	0.45	0.05	0.40	0.50	11%	0	1
Total Words	499	86	412	585	17%	300	680
Different Words	177	23	154	200	13%	120	215
Utterances with Mazes	24	7	16	31	30%	12	41
Utterances with Overlaps	9	5	5	14	51%	0	21
Bound Morphemes Frequency							
Regular Past	4	3	0	7	94%	0	15
Plural	17	8	9	24	48%	4	43
Possessive	2	2	0	3	109%	0	6
Third Person Singular	6	5	2	11	73%	0	19
Present Progressive	4	3	1	6	74%	0	11
Utterance Content							
Personal Pronouns (Total)	77	18	60	95	23%	51	116
(Types)	10	2	8	11	16%	6	12
Total Questions	4	4	0	8	94%	0	17
(WH Total)	2	2	0	5	98%	0	9
(WH Types)	1	1	0	2	78%	0	3
Negatives (Total)	15	6	9	20	40%	6	30
(Types)	6	2	4	7	27%	3	9
Conjunctions (Total)	40	17	23	57	43%	11	99
(Types)	6	1	4	7	22%	3	8
Modals (Total)	5	3	2	8	62%	0	14
(Types)	2	1	1	3	51%	0	4

Variables	Rate 12 Minute Samples						
	Mean	**SD**	**SD–**	**SD+**	**%SD**	**R–**	**R+**
Total Utterances	154	33	122	187	21%	105	224
Complete and Intelligible Utterances	145	31	114	176	21%	95	216
Total Words	709	154	554	863	22%	436	992
Different Words	220	33	187	254	15%	151	281
Mean Length of Utterance (MLU)	5.42	0.85	4.57	6.28	16%	4	7
Between Utterance Pauses	16.54	11.03	5.51	27.58	67%	2	44
Between Utterance Pause Time	1.02	0.84	0.18	1.86	83%	0.1	3.3
Within Utterance Pauses	1.94	2.27	-0.33	4.22	117%	0	9
Within Utterance Pause Time	0.11	0.15	-0.04	0.25	136%	0.0	0.6
Words per Minute	68.35	13.83	54.52	82.18	20%	42	98
Utterances per Minute	12.88	2.71	10.17	15.59	21%	9	19

Content and Rate Summary / 7-Year-Olds

(Conversation N=50)

Variables	Content 100 Utterance Samples						
	Mean	SD	SD–	SD+	%SD	R–	R+
Mean Length of Utterance (MLU)	5.92	0.90	5.02	6.82	15%	4	8
Type Token Ratio	0.45	0.04	0.41	0.49	9%	0	1
Total Words	540	83	457	622	15%	362	705
Different Words	192	19	173	212	10%	155	235
Utterances with Mazes	26	10	16	36	37%	7	54
Utterances with Overlaps	7	6	1	12	85%	0	19
Bound Morphemes Frequency							
Regular Past	5	3	2	8	66%	0	14
Plural	17	6	10	23	37%	6	31
Possessive	2	2	0	4	114%	0	9
Third Person Singular	6	5	2	11	75%	0	20
Present Progressive	4	3	2	7	60%	0	12
Utterance Content							
Personal Pronouns (Total)	81	16	64	97	20%	36	125
(Types)	10	1	8	11	14%	6	12
Total Questions	2	2	0	5	106%	0	11
(WH Total)	1	1	0	2	152%	0	7
(WH Types)	1	1	0	1	120%	0	3
Negatives (Total)	14	6	8	20	43%	3	30
(Types)	6	2	4	8	30%	3	11
Conjunctions (Total)	51	18	33	69	35%	12	102
(Types)	7	1	5	8	20%	4	9
Modals (Total)	5	4	1	9	75%	0	19
(Types)	2	1	1	3	52%	0	6

Variables	Rate 12 Minute Samples						
	Mean	SD	SD–	SD+	%SD	R–	R+
Total Utterances	170	32	138	202	19%	102	232
Complete and Intelligible Utterances	159	29	130	188	18%	96	217
Total Words	858	206	652	1064	24%	420	1478
Different Words	256	37	219	293	14%	164	330
Mean Length of Utterance (MLU)	5.93	0.93	5.00	6.86	16%	4	9
Between Utterance Pauses	13.74	11.66	2.08	25.40	85%	0	59
Between Utterance Pause Time	0.76	0.72	0.04	1.49	95%	0.0	3.2
Within Utterance Pauses	3.10	3.68	-0.58	6.78	119%	0	15
Within Utterance Pause Time	0.18	0.24	-0.06	0.42	133%	0.0	1.1
Words per Minute	83.43	21.47	61.96	104.90	26%	42	139
Utterances per Minute	14.13	2.67	11.47	16.80	19%	9	19

Content and Rate Summary / 9-Year-Olds

(Conversation N=27)

	Content 100 Utterance Samples						
Variables	**Mean**	**SD**	**SD–**	**SD+**	**%SD**	**R–**	**R+**
Mean Length of Utterance (MLU)	6.50	1.06	5.44	7.56	16%	5	8
Type Token Ratio	0.44	0.06	0.38	0.50	14%	0	1
Total Words	592	95	496	687	16%	431	742
Different Words	209	26	183	235	13%	167	278
Utterances with Mazes	23	7	16	30	32%	8	39
Utterances with Overlaps	0	0	0	0	0%	0	0
Bound Morphemes Frequency							
Regular Past	4	3	1	8	74%	0	16
Plural	20	8	11	28	43%	5	44
Possessive	3	2	0	5	94%	0	12
Third Person Singular	6	3	2	9	59%	0	15
Present Progressive	4	3	2	7	60%	0	10
Utterance Content							
Personal Pronouns (Total)	85	16	69	101	19%	41	117
(Types)	9	1	8	11	14%	6	12
Total Questions	2	2	-1	4	127%	0	8
(WH Total)	1	1	0	2	132%	0	3
(WH Types)	0	1	0	1	120%	0	2
Negatives (Total)	11	6	5	17	53%	1	25
(Types)	5	2	3	7	42%	1	10
Conjunctions (Total)	61	23	39	84	37%	27	112
(Types)	8	1	6	9	15%	6	10
Modals (Total)	4	2	2	6	58%	0	9
(Types)	2	1	1	3	48%	0	4

	Rate 12 Minute Samples						
Variables	**Mean**	**SD**	**SD–**	**SD+**	**%SD**	**R–**	**R+**
Total Utterances	181	31	150	212	17%	104	249
Complete and Intelligible Utterances	167	29	138	197	17%	84	233
Total Words	997	256	740	1253	26%	335	1510
Different Words	290	44	246	334	15%	163	373
Mean Length of Utterance (MLU)	6.51	1.09	5.42	7.60	17%	4	8
Between Utterance Pauses	7.70	6.35	1.35	14.06	82%	0	25
Between Utterance Pause Time	0.40	0.44	-0.04	0.83	110%	0.0	2.1
Within Utterance Pauses	1.67	1.82	-0.15	3.49	109%	0	6
Within Utterance Pause Time	0.08	0.09	-0.01	0.17	109%	0.0	0.3
Words per Minute	96.12	25.10	71.02	121.22	26%	40	146
Utterances per Minute	15.11	2.59	12.52	17.70	17%	9	21

Content and Rate Summary / 11-Year-Olds

(Conversation N=27)

Variables	Content 100 Utterance Samples						
	Mean	SD	SD–	SD+	%SD	R–	R+
Mean Length of Utterance (MLU)	7.62	1.94	5.68	9.56	25%	4	12
Type Token Ratio	0.43	0.06	0.37	0.48	14%	0	1
Total Words	693	175	518	868	25%	351	1057
Different Words	229	38	191	267	17%	150	292
Utterances with Mazes	22	9	13	32	41%	6	42
Utterances with Overlaps	7	8	0	15	106%	0	21
Bound Morphemes Frequency							
Regular Past	6	4	2	11	66%	1	18
Plural	20	7	13	28	37%	5	34
Possessive	5	4	0	9	95%	0	18
Third Person Singular	7	5	2	12	67%	1	18
Present Progressive	6	4	2	11	70%	1	20
Utterance Content							
Personal Pronouns (Total)	90	27	63	117	30%	42	134
(Types)	10	1	8	11	15%	6	12
Total Questions	1	2	0	3	119%	0	5
(WH Total)	0	1	0	1	156%	0	2
(WH Types)	0	1	0	1	156%	0	2
Negatives (Total)	14	5	9	19	34%	6	25
(Types)	5	2	4	7	28%	2	9
Conjunctions (Total)	74	31	43	105	42%	17	136
(Types)	8	2	6	10	23%	4	11
Modals (Total)	4	2	2	6	62%	0	11
(Types)	2	1	1	3	59%	0	5

Variables	Rate 12 Minute Samples						
	Mean	SD	SD–	SD+	%SD	R–	R+
Total Utterances	169	38	130	207	23%	92	231
Complete and Intelligible Utterances	158	36	122	194	23%	86	215
Total Words	1112	318	795	1430	29%	293	1619
Different Words	312	61	251	373	19%	126	434
Mean Length of Utterance (MLU)	7.78	1.77	6.00	9.55	23%	4	11
Between Utterance Pauses	8.11	7.69	0.42	15.80	95%	0	30
Between Utterance Pause Time	0.47	0.59	-0.12	1.05	126%	0.0	2.4
Within Utterance Pauses	1.04	1.16	-0.12	2.20	112%	0	4
Within Utterance Pause Time	0.05	0.05	-0.01	0.10	117%	0.0	0.2
Words per Minute	103.86	31.41	72.45	135.27	30%	27	157
Utterances per Minute	14.06	3.18	10.87	17.24	23%	8	19

Content and Rate Summary / 13-Year-Olds

(Conversation N=27)

Variables	Content 100 Utterance Samples						
	Mean	SD	SD–	SD+	%SD	R–	R+
Mean Length of Utterance (MLU)	6.99	1.43	5.56	8.42	21%	5	10
Type Token Ratio	0.43	0.05	0.38	0.48	11%	0	1
Total Words	637	134	503	770	21%	439	900
Different Words	216	31	186	247	14%	166	274
Utterances with Mazes	23	8	14	31	37%	11	39
Utterances with Overlaps	14	7	6	21	54%	2	30
Bound Morphemes Frequency							
Regular Past	4	3	0	7	89%	0	14
Plural	19	5	14	24	28%	7	29
Possessive	1	1	0	2	129%	0	5
Third Person Singular	5	4	2	9	65%	0	15
Present Progressive	7	3	4	10	45%	3	16
Utterance Content							
Personal Pronouns (Total)	93	24	69	117	26%	60	152
(Types)	9	2	8	11	19%	5	12
Total Questions	2	2	0	4	101%	0	8
(WH Total)	1	2	0	3	137%	0	6
(WH Types)	1	1	0	1	110%	0	2
Negatives (Total)	15	6	9	20	38%	6	29
(Types)	5	2	4	7	31%	3	9
Conjunctions (Total)	70	25	45	95	35%	32	132
(Types)	8	2	6	9	21%	5	11
Modals (Total)	4	3	1	7	71%	0	12
(Types)	2	1	1	3	63%	0	5

Variables	Rate 12 Minute Samples						
	Mean	SD	SD–	SD+	%SD	R–	R+
Total Utterances	200	43	157	242	21%	133	333
Complete and Intelligible Utterances	185	38	147	222	20%	129	291
Total Words	1158	297	861	1455	26%	569	1702
Different Words	318	52	266	369	16%	225	464
Mean Length of Utterance (MLU)	6.93	1.37	5.56	8.30	20%	5	10
Between Utterance Pauses	2.96	4.22	-1.26	7.18	142%	0	18
Between Utterance Pause Time	0.21	0.42	-0.21	0.63	200%	0.0	2.1
Within Utterance Pauses	0.59	1.01	-0.42	1.60	170%	0	4
Within Utterance Pause Time	0.02	0.04	0.01	0.06	162%	0.0	0.1
Words per Minute	109.48	29.21	80.27	138.69	27%	53	171
Utterances per Minute	16.64	3.55	13.08	20.19	21%	11	28

Content and Rate Summary / 3-Year-Olds

(Narration N=42)

Variables	Content 100 Utterance Samples						
	Mean	**SD**	**SD–**	**SD+**	**%SD**	**R–**	**R+**
Mean Length of Utterance (MLU)	4.01	0.88	3.12	4.89	22%	2	7
Type Token Ratio	0.45	0.06	0.39	0.51	14%	0	1
Total Words	364	82	283	446	22%	228	608
Different Words	127	23	105	150	18%	83	193
Utterances with Mazes	19	9	10	28	49%	5	36
Utterances with Overlaps	12	5	6	17	46%	2	27

Bound Morphemes Frequency

Regular Past	4	4	-1	8	119%	0	20
Plural	8	5	3	13	66%	0	21
Possessive	3	3	0	6	108%	0	12
Third Person Singular	3	3	0	5	105%	0	11
Present Progressive	7	5	2	12	67%	0	20

Utterance Content

Personal Pronouns (Total)	47	17	30	64	36%	20	83
(Types)	8	1	6	9	18%	5	10
Total Questions	10	7	3	17	73%	0	28
(WH Total)	6	6	1	12	89%	0	22
(WH Types)	2	1	1	4	55%	0	5
Negatives (Total)	12	9	3	20	77%	0	38
(Types)	4	2	2	5	41%	0	7
Conjunctions (Total)	23	19	4	42	82%	1	92
(Types)	3	2	2	5	54%	1	9
Modals (Total)	2	2	0	5	98%	0	9
(Types)	1	1	0	3	78%	0	4

Variables	Rate 12 Minute Samples						
	Mean	**SD**	**SD–**	**SD+**	**%SD**	**R–**	**R+**
Total Utterances	143	34	109	177	24%	82	207
Complete and Intelligible Utterances	121	25	96	146	21%	73	175
Total Words	435	129	306	564	30%	247	818
Different Words	143	31	111	174	22%	97	256
Mean Length of Utterance (MLU)	3.98	0.88	3.10	4.85	22%	3	7
Between Utterance Pauses	30.05	13.56	16.49	43.61	45%	0	58
Between Utterance Pause Time	1.81	1.00	0.81	2.81	55%	0.0	4.2
Within Utterance Pauses	0.76	1.36	-0.60	2.12	178%	0	7
Within Utterance Pause Time	0.03	0.06	-0.03	0.09	194%	0.0	0.3
Words per Minute	45.94	13.26	32.68	59.20	29%	23	77
Utterances per Minute	11.93	2.85	9.08	14.78	24%	7	17

Content and Rate Summary / 4-Year-Olds

(Narration N=30)

	Content 100 Utterance Samples						
Variables	**Mean**	**SD**	**SD–**	**SD+**	**%SD**	**R–**	**R+**
Mean Length of Utterance (MLU)	5.23	1.02	4.21	6.25	20%	3	7
Type Token Ratio	0.43	0.07	0.36	0.50	15%	0	1
Total Words	478	94	383	572	20%	312	659
Different Words	163	23	140	185	14%	117	223
Utterances with Mazes	26	11	15	37	42%	6	47
Utterances with Overlaps	12	5	7	17	46%	2	24
Bound Morphemes Frequency							
Regular Past	6	5	1	11	84%	0	17
Plural	13	7	6	20	56%	3	27
Possessive	3	3	0	6	100%	0	11
Third Person Singular	6	6	0	12	102%	0	27
Present Progressive	4	4	0	8	90%	0	15
Utterance Content							
Personal Pronouns (Total)	64	16	47	80	26%	27	94
(Types)	9	2	7	10	17%	6	12
Total Questions	6	4	2	9	68%	0	15
(WH Total)	3	2	1	5	80%	0	8
(WH Types)	1	1	0	2	66%	0	3
Negatives (Total)	16	8	8	24	51%	1	33
(Types)	5	2	3	7	36%	1	10
Conjunctions (Total)	47	23	24	71	50%	13	106
(Types)	5	1	4	6	24%	3	7
Modals (Total)	4	3	1	7	85%	0	14
(Types)	2	1	1	3	62%	0	5

	Rate 12 Minute Samples						
Variables	**Mean**	**SD**	**SD–**	**SD+**	**%SD**	**R–**	**R+**
Total Utterances	121	32	90	153	26%	71	189
Complete and Intelligible Utterances	109	27	82	136	25%	62	172
Total Words	515	152	362	667	30%	262	862
Different Words	169	35	134	205	21%	106	260
Mean Length of Utterance (MLU)	5.19	0.97	4.22	6.16	19%	3	7
Between Utterance Pauses	17.37	12.17	5.20	29.54	70%	0	43
Between Utterance Pause Time	1.12	0.93	0.19	2.05	83%	0.0	3.7
Within Utterance Pauses	1.80	2.11	-0.31	3.91	117%	0	8
Within Utterance Pause Time	0.09	0.11	-0.02	0.20	117%	0.0	0.4
Words per Minute	53.36	15.92	37.44	69.28	30%	26	86
Utterances per Minute	10.09	2.63	7.46	12.72	26%	6	16

Content and Rate Summary / 5-Year-Olds

(Narration N=28)

Content
100 Utterance Samples

Variables	Mean	SD	SD–	SD+	%SD	R–	R+
Mean Length of Utterance (MLU)	6.06	0.94	5.12	7.00	15%	4	8
Type Token Ratio	0.41	0.07	0.34	0.48	17%	0	1
Total Words	553	91	462	644	16%	392	730
Different Words	178	18	160	197	10%	150	218
Utterances with Mazes	26	10	16	37	38%	10	44
Utterances with Overlaps	10	6	4	17	62%	0	22

Bound Morphemes Frequency

	Mean	SD	SD–	SD+	%SD	R–	R+
Regular Past	8	5	3	14	67%	1	27
Plural	11	5	5	16	49%	3	25
Possessive	7	5	1	12	81%	0	16
Third Person Singular	7	7	-1	14	111%	0	31
Present Progressive	7	5	3	12	66%	0	18

Utterance Content

	Mean	SD	SD–	SD+	%SD	R–	R+
Personal Pronouns (Total)	76	20	57	96	26%	37	109
(Types)	9	1	8	10	13%	7	11
Total Questions	7	5	2	11	66%	0	19
(WH Total)	4	3	1	7	77%	0	10
(WH Types)	2	1	1	3	67%	0	4
Negatives (Total)	16	6	10	22	39%	4	29
(Types)	6	2	4	7	35%	2	9
Conjunctions (Total)	56	27	30	83	47%	21	113
(Types)	6	1	4	7	22%	3	7
Modals (Total)	5	3	1	8	70%	0	15
(Types)	2	1	1	4	51%	0	5

Rate
12 Minute Samples

Variables	Mean	SD	SD–	SD+	%SD	R–	R+
Total Utterances	140	22	118	162	16%	99	189
Complete and Intelligible Utterances	130	22	108	152	17%	93	181
Total Words	709	143	566	852	20%	415	1110
Different Words	208	29	179	237	14%	161	284
Mean Length of Utterance (MLU)	6.03	0.98	5.06	7.01	16%	4	8
Between Utterance Pauses	21.32	11.28	10.04	32.60	53%	4	40
Between Utterance Pause Time	1.27	0.83	0.44	2.09	65%	0.2	3.2
Within Utterance Pauses	2.89	4.18	-1.29	7.08	145%	0	22
Within Utterance Pause Time	0.16	0.27	-0.11	0.43	166%	0.0	1.4
Words per Minute	69.04	13.68	55.36	82.72	20%	40	101
Utterances per Minute	11.66	1.87	9.79	13.53	16%	8	16

Content and Rate Summary / 6-Year-Olds

(Narration N=35)

Variables	Content 100 Utterance Samples						
	Mean	**SD**	**SD–**	**SD+**	**%SD**	**R–**	**R+**
Mean Length of Utterance (MLU)	6.17	1.20	4.97	7.37	19%	4	9
Type Token Ratio	0.41	0.07	0.34	0.47	16%	0	1
Total Words	564	112	453	676	20%	363	792
Different Words	180	26	154	205	14%	139	232
Utterances with Mazes	27	9	18	35	32%	9	40
Utterances with Overlaps	10	5	4	15	58%	0	22
Bound Morphemes Frequency							
Regular Past	11	5	6	16	47%	2	20
Plural	10	5	5	15	46%	3	20
Possessive	5	4	0	9	95%	0	16
Third Person Singular	6	6	0	12	103%	0	25
Present Progressive	6	4	2	11	72%	0	19
Utterance Content							
Personal Pronouns (Total)	82	19	63	100	23%	51	126
(Types)	9	1	8	10	10%	7	11
Total Questions	5	4	1	8	86%	0	15
(WH Total)	3	3	0	6	113%	0	14
(WH Types)	1	1	0	2	95%	0	4
Negatives (Total)	15	7	9	22	44%	3	33
(Types)	6	2	4	7	30%	3	10
Conjunctions (Total)	61	27	34	87	44%	17	122
(Types)	6	1	4	7	26%	2	9
Modals (Total)	5	3	2	8	65%	0	14
(Types)	2	1	1	3	55%	0	4

Variables	Rate 12 Minute Samples						
	Mean	**SD**	**SD–**	**SD+**	**%SD**	**R–**	**R+**
Total Utterances	146	27	119	174	19%	89	203
Complete and Intelligible Utterances	136	26	110	162	19%	84	197
Total Words	774	183	591	956	24%	329	1154
Different Words	217	39	179	256	18%	138	329
Mean Length of Utterance (MLU)	6.24	1.17	5.06	7.41	19%	4	9
Between Utterance Pauses	15.43	10.02	5.41	25.45	65%	2	45
Between Utterance Pause Time	0.92	0.87	0.04	1.79	95%	0.1	4.1
Within Utterance Pauses	3.00	4.39	-1.39	7.39	146%	0	23
Within Utterance Pause Time	0.16	0.24	-0.09	0.40	155%	0.0	1.3
Words per Minute	76.58	16.79	59.79	93.37	22%	30	104
Utterances per Minute	12.35	2.26	10.09	14.62	18%	7	17

Content and Rate Summary / 7-Year-Olds

(Narration N=50)

Variables	Content 100 Utterance Samples						
	Mean	SD	SD–	SD+	%SD	R–	R+
Mean Length of Utterance (MLU)	7.32	1.06	6.26	8.38	15%	5	10
Type Token Ratio	0.38	0.07	0.31	0.45	19%	0	1
Total Words	663	97	566	761	15%	434	880
Different Words	194	20	174	215	10%	161	237
Utterances with Mazes	33	13	20	46	38%	10	75
Utterances with Overlaps	4	4	0	8	101%	0	16

Bound Morphemes Frequency

	Mean	SD	SD–	SD+	%SD	R–	R+
Regular Past	12	7	5	19	61%	0	39
Plural	14	6	8	20	40%	6	34
Possessive	5	4	1	9	83%	0	12
Third Person Singular	10	13	-3	23	132%	0	53
Present Progressive	9	5	3	14	61%	1	26

Utterance Content

	Mean	SD	SD–	SD+	%SD	R–	R+
Personal Pronouns (Total)	90	16	74	106	18%	55	138
(Types)	9	1	8	10	16%	6	12
Total Questions	3	3	1	6	85%	0	14
(WH Total)	2	2	0	4	123%	0	10
(WH Types)	1	1	0	2	98%	0	4
Negatives (Total)	11	4	7	16	39%	2	25
(Types)	5	2	4	7	31%	2	9
Conjunctions (Total)	91	30	61	121	33%	33	160
(Types)	7	1	5	8	19%	4	9
Modals (Total)	5	4	1	8	75%	0	19
(Types)	2	1	1	3	44%	0	4

Variables	Rate 12 Minute Samples						
	Mean	SD	SD–	SD+	%SD	R–	R+
Total Utterances	154	32	122	187	21%	88	270
Complete and Intelligible Utterances	143	30	113	173	21%	85	247
Total Words	928	234	694	1163	25%	426	1582
Different Words	245	41	204	286	17%	157	342
Mean Length of Utterance (MLU)	7.16	1.08	6.08	8.24	15%	5	10
Between Utterance Pauses	12.92	10.21	2.71	23.13	79%	1	44
Between Utterance Pause Time	0.76	0.67	0.09	1.43	88%	0.0	2.9
Within Utterance Pauses	4.46	4.30	0.16	8.76	96%	0	19
Within Utterance Pause Time	0.23	0.22	0.01	0.46	95%	0.0	0.8
Words per Minute	91.87	24.22	67.65	116.09	26%	44	157
Utterances per Minute	12.87	2.69	10.18	15.56	21%	7	23

Content and Rate Summary / 9-Year-Olds

(Narration N=27)

Content
100 Utterance Samples

Variables	Mean	SD	SD–	SD+	%SD	R–	R+
Mean Length of Utterance (MLU)	8.80	1.64	7.17	10.44	19%	6	14
Type Token Ratio	0.33	0.06	0.27	0.38	17%	0	0
Total Words	800	148	653	948	18%	578	1232
Different Words	205	29	176	233	14%	152	264
Utterances with Mazes	31	10	21	40	32%	16	51
Utterances with Overlaps	0	0	0	0	0%	0	0

Bound Morphemes Frequency

Variables	Mean	SD	SD–	SD+	%SD	R–	R+
Regular Past	16	8	8	24	51%	4	37
Plural	17	6	11	23	37%	5	27
Possessive	6	4	2	11	74%	1	14
Third Person Singular	10	11	-1	21	110%	0	48
Present Progressive	11	5	5	16	50%	2	21

Utterance Content

Variables	Mean	SD	SD–	SD+	%SD	R–	R+
Personal Pronouns (Total)	99	19	80	118	19%	63	149
(Types)	9	1	8	10	13%	7	11
Total Questions	4	3	1	7	85%	0	12
(WH Total)	2	2	0	4	115%	0	7
(WH Types)	1	1	0	3	102%	0	4
Negatives (Total)	9	5	4	14	53%	1	20
(Types)	5	2	3	7	41%	1	8
Conjunctions (Total)	108	29	79	136	27%	60	184
(Types)	7	1	5	8	20%	4	9
Modals (Total)	5	4	1	9	80%	0	16
(Types)	2	1	1	3	55%	0	4

Rate
12 Minute Samples

Variables	Mean	SD	SD–	SD+	%SD	R–	R+
Total Utterances	184	35	149	219	19%	110	282
Complete and Intelligible Utterances	171	33	139	204	19%	106	269
Total Words	1312	233	1080	1545	18%	933	1832
Different Words	291	34	256	325	12%	210	380
Mean Length of Utterance (MLU)	8.57	1.61	6.96	10.17	19%	6	14
Between Utterance Pauses	6.04	5.07	0.96	11.11	84%	0	22
Between Utterance Pause Time	0.32	0.28	0.04	0.60	87%	0.0	1.3
Within Utterance Pauses	2.00	2.60	-0.60	4.60	130%	0	10
Within Utterance Pause Time	0.10	0.15	-0.05	0.25	148%	0.0	0.7
Words per Minute	125.94	21.29	104.64	147.23	17%	94	176
Utterances per Minute	15.36	2.92	12.44	18.28	19%	9	24

Content and Rate Summary / 11-Year-Olds

(Narration N=27)

Variables	Content 100 Utterance Samples						
	Mean	**SD**	**SD–**	**SD+**	**%SD**	**R–**	**R+**
Mean Length of Utterance (MLU)	9.83	1.59	8.24	11.42	16%	8	14
Type Token Ratio	0.37	0.04	0.33	0.41	10%	0	0
Total Words	878	138	740	1016	16%	672	1229
Different Words	253	34	219	286	13%	214	383
Utterances with Mazes	38	11	27	49	29%	16	59
Utterances with Overlaps	4	4	-1	8	116%	0	14
Bound Morphemes Frequency							
Regular Past	17	7	9	24	45%	5	33
Plural	23	9	14	33	39%	9	45
Possessive	2	2	0	5	92%	0	9
Third Person Singular	19	18	1	38	93%	0	67
Present Progressive	15	7	7	22	49%	4	30
Utterance Content							
Personal Pronouns (Total)	124	20	103	144	16%	100	190
(Types)	9	1	8	11	11%	6	11
Total Questions	1	2	-1	3	151%	0	8
(WH Total)	0	1	-1	1	211%	0	4
(WH Types)	0	1	0	1	200%	0	3
Negatives (Total)	13	6	7	19	46%	3	32
(Types)	6	2	4	8	34%	1	10
Conjunctions (Total)	118	29	89	148	25%	70	178
(Types)	8	1	7	9	17%	5	10
Modals (Total)	6	5	1	11	79%	0	23
(Types)	2	1	1	4	56%	0	5

Variables	Rate 12 Minute Samples						
	Mean	**SD**	**SD–**	**SD+**	**%SD**	**R–**	**R+**
Total Utterances	167	26	141	193	15%	105	217
Complete and Intelligible Utterances	154	25	129	180	16%	93	206
Total Words	1337	203	1133	1540	15%	681	1639
Different Words	331	48	283	379	14%	205	457
Mean Length of Utterance (MLU)	9.76	1.53	8.23	11.29	16%	7	14
Between Utterance Pauses	5.48	5.09	0.39	10.57	93%	0	19
Between Utterance Pause Time	0.33	0.34	-0.01	0.67	102%	0.0	1.3
Within Utterance Pauses	2.19	3.17	-0.99	5.36	145%	0	14
Within Utterance Pause Time	0.12	0.25	-0.13	0.37	210%	0.0	1.3
Words per Minute	129.50	19.77	109.73	149.28	15%	69	159
Utterances per Minute	13.91	2.13	11.78	16.04	15%	9	18

Content and Rate Summary / 13-Year-Olds

(Narration N=27)

Content
100 Utterance Samples

Variables	Mean	SD	SD–	SD+	%SD	R–	R+
Mean Length of Utterance (MLU)	9.32	1.49	7.83	10.80	16%	7	13
Type Token Ratio	0.36	0.03	0.33	0.40	9%	0	0
Total Words	842	132	710	975	16%	661	1217
Different Words	237	27	210	264	12%	187	284
Utterances with Mazes	33	9	24	42	27%	15	51
Utterances with Overlaps	8	6	2	13	75%	0	21

Bound Morphemes Frequency

	Mean	SD	SD–	SD+	%SD	R–	R+
Regular Past	14	6	7	20	47%	3	32
Plural	20	9	11	28	43%	7	42
Possessive	2	2	0	4	88%	0	8
Third Person Singular	16	12	4	29	75%	1	51
Present Progressive	11	6	5	17	54%	2	23

Utterance Content

	Mean	SD	SD–	SD+	%SD	R–	R+
Personal Pronouns (Total)	123	21	103	144	17%	93	179
(Types)	9	1	8	11	15%	7	11
Total Questions	2	3	-1	4	146%	0	11
(WH Total)	1	1	0	2	132%	0	3
(WH Types)	1	1	0	1	126%	0	2
Negatives (Total)	13	5	8	18	37%	4	27
(Types)	6	2	5	8	28%	3	9
Conjunctions (Total)	108	21	88	129	19%	81	148
(Types)	8	1	6	9	18%	5	11
Modals (Total)	6	4	2	9	62%	0	13
(Types)	2	1	1	3	39%	0	4

Rate
12 Minute Samples

Variables	Mean	SD	SD–	SD+	%SD	R–	R+
Total Utterances	200	46	154	246	23%	129	291
Complete and Intelligible Utterances	180	39	142	219	21%	118	252
Total Words	1443	270	1173	1713	19%	902	1796
Different Words	331	37	294	368	11%	257	393
Mean Length of Utterance (MLU)	8.98	1.50	7.49	10.48	17%	7	13
Between Utterance Pauses	4.41	6.23	-1.82	10.64	141%	0	23
Between Utterance Pause Time	0.22	0.31	-0.10	0.53	145%	0.0	1.1
Within Utterance Pauses	1.30	1.64	-0.34	2.93	126%	0	6
Within Utterance Pause Time	0.05	0.07	-0.02	0.13	133%	0.0	0.3
Words per Minute	139.50	28.74	110.76	168.23	21%	88	195
Utterances per Minute	16.68	3.82	12.85	20.50	23%	11	24

Mean Percentage of Utterances with Mazes by Utterance Length

(100 Utterance Samples)

Conversation

Age Group	\multicolumn{13}{c}{Utterance Length in Morphemes}	Total of Percentages
	1	2	3	4	5	6	7	8	9	10	11	12	13+	
3	3%	10%	16%	21%	27%	26%	28%	26%	30%	15%	21%	12%	28%	16%
4	3%	9%	17%	15%	25%	29%	30%	38%	34%	35%	41%	31%	36%	19%
5	4%	10%	15%	18%	19%	26%	29%	32%	39%	41%	28%	28%	46%	22%
6	4%	9%	16%	19%	23%	27%	32%	37%	33%	42%	48%	41%	57%	24%
7	3%	16%	21%	22%	26%	25%	28%	36%	40%	38%	41%	38%	61%	26%
9	3%	4%	5%	13%	22%	25%	31%	33%	32%	31%	35%	40%	52%	23%
11	2%	7%	5%	13%	16%	20%	24%	25%	24%	33%	36%	31%	45%	22%
13	3%	5%	9%	10%	25%	24%	24%	22%	40%	28%	36%	32%	47%	23%

Narration

Age Group	\multicolumn{13}{c}{Utterance Length in Morphemes}	Total of Percentages
	1	2	3	4	5	6	7	8	9	10	11	12	13+	
3	2%	13%	16%	21%	26%	29%	35%	37%	29%	29%	26%	34%	31%	19%
4	2%	12%	19%	27%	23%	27%	42%	43%	50%	47%	48%	42%	56%	26%
5	3%	8%	14%	14%	25%	28%	32%	35%	42%	49%	46%	40%	58%	26%
6	4%	13%	11%	20%	28%	23%	30%	40%	36%	36%	43%	38%	55%	27%
7	5%	18%	20%	24%	26%	35%	35%	41%	42%	48%	44%	49%	55%	33%
9	1%	8%	11%	7%	19%	26%	33%	32%	29%	36%	33%	36%	50%	30%
11	3%	11%	19%	12%	24%	30%	32%	41%	37%	37%	46%	52%	61%	38%
13	2%	6%	21%	20%	19%	25%	27%	25%	36%	37%	44%	49%	59%	33%

Word List Summary / 3-Year-Olds
(Conversation: 100 Utterance Samples N=42)

Questions

	Mean	SD	SD–	SD+	%SD	R–	R+
How	0.31	0.84	-0.53	1.15	272%	0	4
What	4.26	4.07	0.19	8.33	96%	0	16
When	0.14	0.65	-0.50	0.79	453%	0	4
Where	0.95	1.64	-0.68	2.59	172%	0	7
Which	0.10	0.37	-0.27	0.47	389%	0	2
Who	0.52	0.86	-0.34	1.39	165%	0	3
Whose	0.00	0.00	0.00	0.00	0%	0	0
Why	0.74	1.48	-0.74	2.22	201%	0	6

Conjunctions

	Mean	SD	SD–	SD+	%SD	R–	R+
After	0.10	0.37	-0.27	0.47	389%	0	2
And	7.50	5.08	2.42	12.58	68%	0	19
As	0.05	0.22	-0.17	0.26	453%	0	1
Because	1.07	1.47	-0.40	2.54	137%	0	5
But	0.95	1.21	-0.26	2.16	127%	0	5
If	0.05	0.22	-0.17	0.26	453%	0	1
Or	0.26	0.59	-0.32	0.85	224%	0	2
Since	0.00	0.00	0.00	0.00	0%	0	0
So	0.33	0.61	-0.28	0.94	183%	0	2
Then	1.33	1.97	-0.64	3.30	148%	0	8
Until	0.00	0.00	0.00	0.00	0%	0	0
While	0.00	0.00	0.00	0.00	0%	0	0

Negatives

	Mean	SD	SD–	SD+	%SD	R–	R+
Ain't	0.02	0.15	-0.13	0.18	648%	0	1
Are/n't	0.02	0.15	-0.13	0.18	648%	0	1
Can/'t	1.02	1.35	-0.33	2.38	132%	0	5
Could/n't	0.02	0.15	-0.13	0.18	648%	0	1
Did/n't	0.64	1.01	-0.36	1.65	157%	0	4
Does/n't	0.62	1.06	-0.44	1.68	171%	0	5
Don't	3.05	3.04	0.01	6.08	100%	0	12
Had/n't	0.00	0.00	0.00	0.00	0%	0	0
Has/n't	0.00	0.00	0.00	0.00	0%	0	0
Have/n't	0.02	0.15	-0.13	0.18	648%	0	1
Is/n't	0.07	0.26	-0.19	0.33	365%	0	1
Might/n't	0.00	0.00	0.00	0.00	0%	0	0
Must/n't	0.00	0.00	0.00	0.00	0%	0	0
No	4.05	3.08	0.96	7.13	76%	0	15
Nope	0.36	0.82	-0.46	1.18	230%	0	4
Not	1.07	1.35	-0.28	2.42	126%	0	5
Should/n't	0.00	0.00	0.00	0.00	0%	0	0
Uhuh	0.50	1.09	-0.59	1.59	218%	0	5
Was/n't	0.07	0.34	-0.27	0.41	478%	0	2
Were/n't	0.00	0.00	0.00	0.00	0%	0	0
Won't	0.05	0.22	-0.17	0.26	453%	0	1
Would/n't	0.00	0.00	0.00	0.00	0%	0	0

Modals

	Mean	SD	SD–	SD+	%SD	R–	R+
Can	2.71	2.71	0.01	5.42	100%	0	11
Could	0.40	1.89	-1.48	2.29	466%	0	12
May	0.00	0.00	0.00	0.00	0%	0	0
Might	0.05	0.22	-0.17	0.26	453%	0	1
Must	0.00	0.00	0.00	0.00	0%	0	0
Shall	0.00	0.00	0.00	0.00	0%	0	0
Should	0.33	0.69	-0.35	1.02	206%	0	3
Will	0.40	0.73	-0.33	1.14	181%	0	3
Would	0.02	0.15	-0.13	0.18	648%	0	1

Pronouns

Reflexive

	Mean	SD	SD–	SD+	%SD	R–	R+
Herself	0.00	0.00	0.00	0.00	0%	0	0
Himself	0.00	0.00	0.00	0.00	0%	0	0
Itself	0.00	0.00	0.00	0.00	0%	0	0
Myself	0.07	0.26	-0.19	0.33	365%	0	1
Ourselves	0.00	0.00	0.00	0.00	0%	0	0
Themselves	0.00	0.00	0.00	0.00	0%	0	0
Yourself	0.02	0.15	-0.13	0.18	648%	0	1
Yourselves	0.00	0.00	0.00	0.00	0%	0	0

Demonstrative

	Mean	SD	SD–	SD+	%SD	R–	R+
That	5.07	2.97	2.11	8.04	58%	0	14
These	1.76	2.59	-0.83	4.35	147%	0	15
This	8.64	5.59	3.05	14.23	65%	0	23
Those	0.48	1.06	-0.59	1.54	224%	0	5

Quantifying

	Mean	SD	SD–	SD+	%SD	R–	R+
Enough	0.05	0.22	-0.17	0.26	453%	0	1
Few	0.00	0.00	0.00	0.00	0%	0	0
Little	0.74	1.33	-0.59	2.06	180%	0	5
Many	0.05	0.31	-0.26	0.36	648%	0	2
Much	0.07	0.26	-0.19	0.33	365%	0	1
One	4.17	3.94	0.23	8.10	95%	0	19
Several	0.00	0.00	0.00	0.00	0%	0	0

Relative

	Mean	SD	SD–	SD+	%SD	R–	R+
What	0.52	1.04	-0.52	1.57	199%	0	4
Whatever	0.00	0.00	0.00	0.00	0%	0	0
Which	0.00	0.00	0.00	0.00	0%	0	0
Whichever	0.02	0.15	-0.13	0.18	648%	0	1
Who	0.07	0.26	-0.19	0.33	365%	0	1
Whoever	0.00	0.00	0.00	0.00	0%	0	0
Whom	0.00	0.00	0.00	0.00	0%	0	0
Whose	0.00	0.00	0.00	0.00	0%	0	0

Universal

	Mean	SD	SD–	SD+	%SD	R–	R+
All	1.02	1.18	-0.16	2.20	115%	0	4
Both	0.12	0.45	-0.33	0.57	380%	0	2
Each	0.00	0.00	0.00	0.00	0%	0	0
Every	0.00	0.00	0.00	0.00	0%	0	0
Everybody	0.02	0.15	-0.13	0.18	648%	0	1
Everyone	0.00	0.00	0.00	0.00	0%	0	0
Everything	0.07	0.46	-0.39	0.53	648%	0	3
Everywhere	0.00	0.00	0.00	0.00	0%	0	0

Possessive

	Mean	SD	SD–	SD+	%SD	R–	R+
Her	0.48	0.80	-0.33	1.28	169%	0	3
Hers	0.00	0.00	0.00	0.00	0%	0	0
His	0.69	1.07	-0.38	1.76	155%	0	4
Its	0.00	0.00	0.00	0.00	0%	0	0
Mine	0.31	0.68	-0.37	0.99	220%	0	3
My	5.81	4.73	1.08	10.54	81%	0	16
Our	0.24	0.58	-0.34	0.81	242%	0	2
Ours	0.00	0.00	0.00	0.00	0%	0	0
Their	0.17	0.49	-0.32	0.66	294%	0	2
Theirs	0.00	0.00	0.00	0.00	0%	0	0
Your	0.43	0.86	-0.43	1.29	201%	0	3
Yours	0.05	0.22	-0.17	0.26	453%	0	1

Personal

	Mean	SD	SD–	SD+	%SD	R–	R+
He	3.60	4.20	-0.60	7.79	117%	0	19
Her	0.48	0.80	-0.33	1.28	169%	0	3
Him	1.19	2.13	-0.94	3.32	179%	0	9
I	18.19	8.77	9.42	26.96	48%	5	39
It	8.52	5.14	3.38	13.67	60%	2	22
Me	1.90	2.09	-0.19	4.00	110%	0	9
She	0.88	1.31	-0.43	2.19	149%	0	4
Them	1.21	1.39	-0.17	2.60	114%	0	6
They	1.50	1.92	-0.42	3.42	128%	0	8
Us	0.10	0.30	-0.20	0.39	312%	0	1
We	2.71	3.48	-0.77	6.19	128%	0	17
You	3.67	3.55	0.11	7.22	97%	0	14

Partitive

	Mean	SD	SD–	SD+	%SD	R–	R+
Any	0.26	0.73	-0.47	1.00	280%	0	3
Anybody	0.00	0.00	0.00	0.00	0%	0	0
Anyone	0.00	0.00	0.00	0.00	0%	0	0
Anything	0.05	0.22	-0.17	0.26	453%	0	1
Anywhere	0.00	0.00	0.00	0.00	0%	0	0
Either	0.07	0.26	-0.19	0.33	365%	0	1
Neither	0.00	0.00	0.00	0.00	0%	0	0
Nobody	0.00	0.00	0.00	0.00	0%	0	0
None	0.02	0.15	-0.13	0.18	648%	0	1
No one	0.00	0.00	0.00	0.00	0%	0	0
Nothing	0.57	2.10	-1.53	2.67	367%	0	13
Some	1.71	2.14	-0.43	3.86	125%	0	11
Somebody	0.21	0.52	-0.31	0.73	243%	0	2
Someone	0.05	0.31	-0.26	0.36	648%	0	2
Someplace	0.00	0.00	0.00	0.00	0%	0	0
Something	0.36	0.66	-0.30	1.01	184%	0	2

Word List Summary / 4-Year-Olds
(Conversation: 100 Utterance Samples N=30)

Questions

	Mean	SD	SD–	SD+	%SD	R–	R+
How	0.20	0.48	-0.28	0.68	242%	0	2
What	2.37	2.25	0.12	4.62	95%	0	8
When	0.20	0.55	-0.35	0.75	275%	0	2
Where	0.23	0.57	-0.33	0.80	244%	0	2
Which	0.07	0.25	-0.19	0.32	381%	0	1
Who	0.10	0.31	-0.21	0.41	305%	0	1
Whose	0.00	0.00	0.00	0.00	0%	0	0
Why	0.40	0.50	-0.10	0.90	125%	0	1

Conjunctions

	Mean	SD	SD–	SD+	%SD	R–	R+
After	0.00	0.00	0.00	0.00	0%	0	0
And	13.23	10.78	2.45	24.02	81%	2	47
As	0.07	0.37	-0.30	0.43	548%	0	2
Because	3.27	2.84	0.43	6.11	87%	0	11
But	3.47	3.09	0.37	6.56	89%	0	9
If	0.63	1.22	-0.58	1.85	192%	0	5
Or	0.27	0.64	-0.37	0.91	240%	0	2
Since	0.03	0.18	-0.15	0.22	548%	0	1
So	0.77	1.10	-0.34	1.87	144%	0	4
Then	2.10	3.54	-1.44	5.64	168%	0	17
Until	0.10	0.31	-0.21	0.41	305%	0	1
While	0.03	0.18	-0.15	0.22	548%	0	1

Negatives

	Mean	SD	SD–	SD+	%SD	R–	R+
Ain't	0.00	0.00	0.00	0.00	0%	0	0
Are/n't	0.07	0.37	-0.30	0.43	548%	0	2
Can't	0.73	1.11	-0.38	1.85	152%	0	4
Could/n't	0.00	0.00	0.00	0.00	0%	0	0
Did/n't	0.57	0.90	-0.33	1.46	158%	0	3
Does/n't	1.00	1.26	-0.26	2.26	126%	0	5
Don't	3.17	3.10	0.07	6.26	98%	0	11
Had/n't	0.00	0.00	0.00	0.00	0%	0	0
Has/n't	0.00	0.00	0.00	0.00	0%	0	0
Have/n't	0.00	0.00	0.00	0.00	0%	0	0
Is/n't	0.07	0.25	-0.19	0.32	381%	0	1
Might/n't	0.00	0.00	0.00	0.00	0%	0	0
Must/n't	0.00	0.00	0.00	0.00	0%	0	0
No	5.43	3.02	2.41	8.46	56%	0	12
Nope	0.20	0.92	-0.72	1.12	462%	0	5
Not	1.23	1.10	0.13	2.34	90%	0	4
Should/n't	0.00	0.00	0.00	0.00	0%	0	0
Uhuh	0.93	1.23	-0.30	2.16	132%	0	4
Was/n't	0.07	0.25	-0.19	0.32	381%	0	1
Were/n't	0.00	0.00	0.00	0.00	0%	0	0
Won't	0.23	0.77	-0.54	1.01	332%	0	4
Would/n't	0.07	0.37	-0.30	0.43	548%	0	2

Modals

	Mean	SD	SD–	SD+	%SD	R–	R+
Can	2.47	2.15	0.32	4.61	87%	0	7
Could	0.50	0.73	-0.23	1.23	146%	0	2
May	0.00	0.00	0.00	0.00	0%	0	0
Might	0.20	0.55	-0.35	0.75	275%	0	2
Must	0.00	0.00	0.00	0.00	0%	0	0
Shall	0.00	0.00	0.00	0.00	0%	0	0
Should	0.20	0.48	-0.28	0.68	242%	0	2
Will	0.33	0.61	-0.27	0.94	182%	0	2
Would	0.40	0.81	-0.41	1.21	203%	0	3

Pronouns

Reflexive

	Mean	SD	SD–	SD+	%SD	R–	R+
Herself	0.00	0.00	0.00	0.00	0%	0	0
Himself	0.00	0.00	0.00	0.00	0%	0	0
Itself	0.00	0.00	0.00	0.00	0%	0	0
Myself	0.00	0.00	0.00	0.00	0%	0	0
Ourselves	0.00	0.00	0.00	0.00	0%	0	0
Themselves	0.00	0.00	0.00	0.00	0%	0	0
Yourself	0.00	0.00	0.00	0.00	0%	0	0
Yourselves	0.00	0.00	0.00	0.00	0%	0	0

Demonstrative

	Mean	SD	SD–	SD+	%SD	R–	R+
That	4.93	3.48	1.45	8.42	71%	0	16
These	0.53	0.90	-0.37	1.43	169%	0	4
This	4.60	4.00	0.60	8.60	87%	0	14
Those	0.67	0.84	-0.18	1.51	127%	0	3

Quantifying

	Mean	SD	SD–	SD+	%SD	R–	R+
Enough	0.10	0.40	-0.30	0.50	403%	0	2
Few	0.00	0.00	0.00	0.00	0%	0	0
Little	1.37	1.85	-0.48	3.21	135%	0	9
Many	0.23	0.68	-0.45	0.91	291%	0	3
Much	0.13	0.57	-0.44	0.70	429%	0	3
One	4.03	3.62	0.41	7.66	90%	0	13
Several	0.00	0.00	0.00	0.00	0%	0	0

Relative

	Mean	SD	SD–	SD+	%SD	R–	R+
What	0.73	1.08	-0.35	1.81	147%	0	4
Whatever	0.03	0.18	-0.15	0.22	548%	0	1
Which	0.17	0.59	-0.43	0.76	355%	0	3
Whichever	0.00	0.00	0.00	0.00	0%	0	0
Who	0.17	0.53	-0.36	0.70	318%	0	2
Whoever	0.00	0.00	0.00	0.00	0%	0	0
Whom	0.00	0.00	0.00	0.00	0%	0	0
Whose	0.00	0.00	0.00	0.00	0%	0	0

Universal

	Mean	SD	SD–	SD+	%SD	R–	R+
All	1.30	1.42	-0.12	2.72	109%	0	5
Both	0.00	0.00	0.00	0.00	0%	0	0
Each	0.03	0.18	-0.15	0.22	548%	0	1
Every	0.13	0.35	-0.21	0.48	259%	0	1
Everybody	0.00	0.00	0.00	0.00	0%	0	0
Everyone	0.07	0.25	-0.19	0.32	381%	0	1
Everything	0.13	0.35	-0.21	0.48	259%	0	1
Everywhere	0.03	0.18	-0.15	0.22	548%	0	1

Possessive

	Mean	SD	SD–	SD+	%SD	R–	R+
Her	1.00	1.46	-0.46	2.46	146%	0	6
Hers	0.07	0.37	-0.30	0.43	548%	0	2
His	1.07	1.68	-0.61	2.75	158%	0	7
Its	0.00	0.00	0.00	0.00	0%	0	0
Mine	0.70	1.39	-0.69	2.09	199%	0	6
My	5.97	3.95	2.01	9.92	66%	0	19
Our	0.37	0.56	-0.19	0.92	152%	0	2
Ours	0.00	0.00	0.00	0.00	0%	0	0
Their	0.33	1.15	-0.82	1.49	346%	0	5
Theirs	0.00	0.00	0.00	0.00	0%	0	0
Your	0.50	0.90	-0.40	1.40	180%	0	4
Yours	0.27	0.58	-0.32	0.85	219%	0	2

Personal

	Mean	SD	SD–	SD+	%SD	R–	R+
He	4.53	4.76	-0.23	9.29	105%	0	18
Her	1.00	1.46	-0.46	2.46	146%	0	6
Him	0.77	1.04	-0.27	1.81	136%	0	4
I	20.93	8.77	12.16	29.71	42%	5	42
It	10.63	4.87	5.76	15.51	46%	3	20
Me	2.73	2.30	0.43	5.04	84%	0	9
She	2.00	2.68	-0.68	4.68	134%	0	9
Them	1.90	3.08	-1.18	4.98	162%	0	16
They	2.50	3.05	-0.55	5.55	122%	0	13
Us	0.30	0.99	-0.69	1.29	329%	0	5
We	3.17	3.29	-0.12	6.46	104%	0	14
You	6.60	4.43	2.17	11.03	67%	0	21

Partitive

	Mean	SD	SD–	SD+	%SD	R–	R+
Any	0.40	0.77	-0.37	1.17	193%	0	3
Anybody	0.00	0.00	0.00	0.00	0%	0	0
Anyone	0.03	0.18	-0.15	0.22	548%	0	1
Anything	0.03	0.18	-0.15	0.22	548%	0	1
Anywhere	0.00	0.00	0.00	0.00	0%	0	0
Either	0.00	0.00	0.00	0.00	0%	0	0
Neither	0.00	0.00	0.00	0.00	0%	0	0
Nobody	0.00	0.00	0.00	0.00	0%	0	0
None	0.03	0.18	-0.15	0.22	548%	0	1
No one	0.00	0.00	0.00	0.00	0%	0	0
Nothing	0.03	0.18	-0.15	0.22	548%	0	1
Some	1.60	1.98	-0.38	3.58	123%	0	7
Somebody	0.17	0.46	-0.29	0.63	277%	0	2
Someone	0.20	0.55	-0.35	0.75	275%	0	2
Someplace	0.00	0.00	0.00	0.00	0%	0	0
Something	0.30	0.60	-0.30	0.90	199%	0	2

Word List Summary / 5-Year-Olds

(Conversation: 100 Utterance Samples N=28)

Questions

Questions	Mean	SD	SD–	SD+	%SD	R–	R+
How	0.68	0.94	-0.27	1.62	139%	0	3
What	2.75	2.85	-0.10	5.60	104%	0	11
When	0.07	0.26	-0.19	0.33	367%	0	1
Where	0.14	0.45	-0.31	0.59	314%	0	2
Which	0.00	0.00	0.00	0.00	0%	0	0
Who	0.36	0.83	-0.47	1.18	231%	0	3
Whose	0.04	0.19	-0.15	0.22	529%	0	1
Why	0.11	0.31	-0.21	0.42	294%	0	1

Conjunctions

Conjunctions	Mean	SD	SD–	SD+	%SD	R–	R+
After	0.50	0.92	-0.42	1.42	185%	0	3
And	23.21	13.51	9.71	36.72	58%	2	56
As	0.32	0.61	-0.29	0.93	190%	0	2
Because	3.50	2.41	1.09	5.91	69%	0	9
But	4.82	3.72	1.10	8.54	77%	0	18
If	1.29	1.84	-0.56	3.13	143%	0	5
Or	1.21	1.13	0.08	2.35	93%	0	4
Since	0.14	0.36	-0.21	0.50	249%	0	1
So	1.86	1.43	0.42	3.29	77%	0	5
Then	4.75	4.16	0.59	8.91	88%	0	17
Until	0.11	0.31	-0.21	0.42	294%	0	1
While	0.14	0.45	-0.31	0.59	314%	0	2

Negatives

Negatives	Mean	SD	SD–	SD+	%SD	R–	R+
Ain't	0.04	0.19	-0.15	0.22	529%	0	1
Are/n't	0.04	0.19	-0.15	0.22	529%	0	1
Can/'t	0.75	0.84	-0.09	1.59	113%	0	3
Could/n't	0.14	0.45	-0.31	0.59	314%	0	2
Did/n't	1.18	1.22	-0.04	2.40	103%	0	4
Does/n't	0.79	1.07	-0.28	1.85	136%	0	3
Don't	4.50	3.32	1.18	7.82	74%	0	11
Had/n't	0.00	0.00	0.00	0.00	0%	0	0
Has/n't	0.00	0.00	0.00	0.00	0%	0	0
Have/n't	0.00	0.00	0.00	0.00	0%	0	0
Is/n't	0.14	0.36	-0.21	0.50	249%	0	1
Might/n't	0.00	0.00	0.00	0.00	0%	0	0
Must/n't	0.00	0.00	0.00	0.00	0%	0	0
No	2.43	2.06	0.37	4.49	85%	0	6
Nope	0.18	0.48	-0.30	0.65	266%	0	2
Not	1.61	1.55	0.06	3.15	96%	0	5
Should/n't	0.00	0.00	0.00	0.00	0%	0	0
Uhuh	0.61	1.03	-0.42	1.64	170%	0	4
Was/n't	0.21	0.42	-0.20	0.63	195%	0	1
Were/n't	0.00	0.00	0.00	0.00	0%	0	0
Won't	0.14	0.36	-0.21	0.50	249%	0	1
Would/n't	0.00	0.00	0.00	0.00	0%	0	0

Modals

Modals	Mean	SD	SD–	SD+	%SD	R–	R+
Can	2.79	1.97	0.82	4.76	71%	0	7
Could	1.00	1.47	-0.47	2.47	147%	0	5
May	0.00	0.00	0.00	0.00	0%	0	0
Might	0.39	0.79	-0.39	1.18	200%	0	3
Must	0.07	0.38	-0.31	0.45	529%	0	2
Shall	0.00	0.00	0.00	0.00	0%	0	0
Should	0.04	0.19	-0.15	0.22	529%	0	1
Will	0.50	0.92	-0.42	1.42	185%	0	4
Would	0.82	1.59	-0.77	2.41	193%	0	7

Pronouns

Reflexive

Reflexive	Mean	SD	SD–	SD+	%SD	R–	R+
Herself	0.00	0.00	0.00	0.00	0%	0	0
Himself	0.04	0.19	-0.15	0.22	529%	0	1
Itself	0.00	0.00	0.00	0.00	0%	0	0
Myself	0.00	0.00	0.00	0.00	0%	0	0
Ourselves	0.00	0.00	0.00	0.00	0%	0	0
Themselves	0.00	0.00	0.00	0.00	0%	0	0
Yourself	0.00	0.00	0.00	0.00	0%	0	0
Yourselves	0.00	0.00	0.00	0.00	0%	0	0

Demonstrative

Demonstrative	Mean	SD	SD–	SD+	%SD	R–	R+
That	6.79	4.69	2.10	11.47	69%	0	19
These	0.96	1.88	-0.91	2.84	194%	0	9
This	6.39	7.15	-0.75	13.54	112%	0	32
Those	0.75	1.67	-0.92	2.42	223%	0	8

Quantifying

Quantifying	Mean	SD	SD–	SD+	%SD	R–	R+
Enough	0.04	0.19	-0.15	0.22	529%	0	1
Few	0.00	0.00	0.00	0.00	0%	0	0
Little	2.29	1.88	0.40	4.17	82%	0	7
Many	0.21	0.50	-0.28	0.71	233%	0	2
Much	0.18	0.39	-0.21	0.57	218%	0	1
One	5.21	3.56	1.65	8.78	68%	0	13
Several	0.00	0.00	0.00	0.00	0%	0	0

Relative

Relative	Mean	SD	SD–	SD+	%SD	R–	R+
What	1.39	1.55	-0.15	2.94	111%	0	5
Whatever	0.11	0.31	-0.21	0.42	294%	0	1
Which	0.21	0.50	-0.28	0.71	233%	0	2
Whichever	0.00	0.00	0.00	0.00	0%	0	0
Who	0.25	0.59	-0.34	0.84	234%	0	2
Whoever	0.18	0.48	-0.30	0.65	266%	0	2
Whom	0.00	0.00	0.00	0.00	0%	0	0
Whose	0.07	0.26	-0.19	0.33	367%	0	1

Universal

Universal	Mean	SD	SD–	SD+	%SD	R–	R+
All	1.79	2.13	-0.35	3.92	119%	0	9
Both	0.29	0.66	-0.37	0.94	231%	0	3
Each	0.21	0.69	-0.47	0.90	320%	0	3
Every	0.04	0.19	-0.15	0.22	529%	0	1
Everybody	0.04	0.19	-0.15	0.22	529%	0	1
Everyone	0.04	0.19	-0.15	0.22	529%	0	1
Everything	0.11	0.42	-0.31	0.52	389%	0	2
Everywhere	0.00	0.00	0.00	0.00	0%	0	0

Possessive

Possessive	Mean	SD	SD–	SD+	%SD	R–	R+
Her	1.61	2.54	-0.94	4.15	158%	0	10
Hers	0.00	0.00	0.00	0.00	0%	0	0
His	1.86	2.27	-0.42	4.13	122%	0	10
Its	0.00	0.00	0.00	0.00	0%	0	0
Mine	0.07	0.26	-0.19	0.33	367%	0	1
My	9.46	7.01	2.46	16.47	74%	0	24
Our	1.89	1.81	0.08	3.71	96%	0	6
Ours	0.04	0.19	-0.15	0.22	529%	0	1
Their	0.57	0.92	-0.35	1.49	161%	0	3
Theirs	0.00	0.00	0.00	0.00	0%	0	0
Your	0.46	0.74	-0.28	1.21	160%	0	2
Yours	0.04	0.19	-0.15	0.22	529%	0	1

Personal

Personal	Mean	SD	SD–	SD+	%SD	R–	R+
He	5.75	4.36	1.39	10.11	76%	0	19
Her	1.61	2.54	-0.94	4.15	158%	0	10
Him	2.46	2.83	-0.37	5.30	115%	0	10
I	23.61	7.45	16.16	31.05	32%	7	41
It	12.64	5.84	6.80	18.49	46%	2	24
Me	3.54	3.93	-0.39	7.47	111%	0	14
She	5.04	5.01	0.03	10.04	99%	0	18
Them	2.82	2.45	0.37	5.27	87%	0	9
They	3.50	3.31	0.19	6.81	94%	0	17
Us	0.39	0.88	-0.48	1.27	223%	0	4
We	9.32	6.67	2.65	15.99	72%	1	24
You	10.64	7.51	3.13	18.15	71%	1	24

Partitive

Partitive	Mean	SD	SD–	SD+	%SD	R–	R+
Any	0.61	0.79	-0.18	1.39	129%	0	2
Anybody	0.00	0.00	0.00	0.00	0%	0	0
Anyone	0.00	0.00	0.00	0.00	0%	0	0
Anything	0.21	0.63	-0.42	0.84	294%	0	3
Anywhere	0.04	0.19	-0.15	0.22	529%	0	1
Either	0.00	0.00	0.00	0.00	0%	0	0
Neither	0.00	0.00	0.00	0.00	0%	0	0
Nobody	0.00	0.00	0.00	0.00	0%	0	0
None	0.04	0.19	-0.15	0.22	529%	0	1
No one	0.00	0.00	0.00	0.00	0%	0	0
Nothing	0.11	0.57	-0.46	0.67	529%	0	3
Some	2.21	2.28	-0.07	4.50	103%	0	10
Somebody	0.07	0.38	-0.31	0.45	529%	0	2
Someone	0.14	0.36	-0.21	0.50	249%	0	1
Someplace	0.00	0.00	0.00	0.00	0%	0	0
Something	0.82	1.12	-0.30	1.95	137%	0	5

Word List Summary / 6-Year-Olds

(Conversation: 100 Utterance Samples N=35)

Questions	Mean	SD	SD-	SD+	%SD	R-	R+
How	0.20	0.47	-0.27	0.67	236%	0	2
What	1.54	1.80	-0.26	3.35	117%	0	7
When	0.11	0.40	-0.29	0.52	353%	0	2
Where	0.14	0.36	-0.21	0.50	249%	0	1
Which	0.17	0.45	-0.28	0.62	264%	0	2
Who	0.09	0.28	-0.20	0.37	331%	0	1
Whose	0.00	0.00	0.00	0.00	0%	0	0
Why	0.09	0.37	-0.29	0.46	436%	0	2

Conjunctions	Mean	SD	SD-	SD+	%SD	R-	R+
After	0.37	0.69	-0.32	1.06	186%	0	3
And	24.46	11.67	12.79	36.12	48%	5	57
As	0.11	0.40	-0.29	0.52	353%	0	2
Because	3.03	2.71	0.32	5.73	89%	0	10
But	4.06	2.84	1.22	6.90	70%	0	12
If	0.83	1.18	-0.35	2.00	142%	0	6
Or	0.91	1.38	-0.47	2.29	151%	0	7
Since	0.00	0.00	0.00	0.00	0%	0	0
So	1.51	2.24	-0.73	3.76	148%	0	10
Then	4.80	5.56	-0.76	10.36	116%	0	28
Until	0.09	0.28	-0.20	0.37	331%	0	1
While	0.09	0.28	-0.20	0.37	331%	0	1

Negatives	Mean	SD	SD-	SD+	%SD	R-	R+
Ain't	0.09	0.37	-0.29	0.46	436%	0	2
Are/n't	0.11	0.40	-0.29	0.52	353%	0	2
Can't	1.29	1.27	0.01	2.56	99%	0	5
Could/n't	0.17	0.51	-0.34	0.69	300%	0	2
Did/n't	1.03	1.29	-0.27	2.32	126%	0	6
Does/n't	0.80	1.16	-0.36	1.96	145%	0	5
Don't	4.51	2.77	1.75	7.28	61%	0	11
Had/n't	0.00	0.00	0.00	0.00	0%	0	0
Has/n't	0.00	0.00	0.00	0.00	0%	0	0
Have/n't	0.00	0.00	0.00	0.00	0%	0	0
Is/n't	0.06	0.24	-0.18	0.29	412%	0	1
Might/n't	0.00	0.00	0.00	0.00	0%	0	0
Must/n't	0.00	0.00	0.00	0.00	0%	0	0
No	3.11	2.48	0.63	5.60	80%	0	9
Nope	0.06	0.24	-0.18	0.29	412%	0	1
Not	1.43	1.65	-0.22	3.08	116%	0	8
Should/n't	0.00	0.00	0.00	0.00	0%	0	0
Uhuh	1.34	2.18	-0.84	3.52	162%	0	11
Was/n't	0.23	0.43	-0.20	0.65	186%	0	1
Were/n't	0.00	0.00	0.00	0.00	0%	0	0
Won't	0.31	0.72	-0.40	1.03	229%	0	3
Would/n't	0.11	0.40	-0.29	0.52	353%	0	2

Modals	Mean	SD	SD-	SD+	%SD	R-	R+
Can	3.46	2.28	1.18	5.74	66%	0	11
Could	0.46	0.89	-0.43	1.34	194%	0	4
May	0.03	0.17	-0.14	0.20	592%	0	1
Might	0.14	0.43	-0.29	0.57	301%	0	2
Must	0.00	0.00	0.00	0.00	0%	0	0
Shall	0.00	0.00	0.00	0.00	0%	0	0
Should	0.14	0.36	-0.21	0.50	249%	0	1
Will	0.23	0.60	-0.37	0.83	262%	0	2
Would	0.40	0.81	-0.41	1.21	203%	0	4

Pronouns

Reflexive	Mean	SD	SD-	SD+	%SD	R-	R+
Herself	0.03	0.17	-0.14	0.20	592%	0	1
Himself	0.00	0.00	0.00	0.00	0%	0	0
Itself	0.03	0.17	-0.14	0.20	592%	0	1
Myself	0.11	0.32	-0.21	0.44	282%	0	1
Ourselves	0.00	0.00	0.00	0.00	0%	0	0
Themselves	0.00	0.00	0.00	0.00	0%	0	0
Yourself	0.00	0.00	0.00	0.00	0%	0	0
Yourselves	0.00	0.00	0.00	0.00	0%	0	0

Demonstrative	Mean	SD	SD-	SD+	%SD	R-	R+
That	7.60	3.98	3.62	11.58	52%	1	17
These	0.54	1.09	-0.55	1.64	202%	0	4
This	3.29	3.74	-0.45	7.02	114%	0	20
Those	0.51	0.74	-0.23	1.26	144%	0	3

Quantifying	Mean	SD	SD-	SD+	%SD	R-	R+
Enough	0.06	0.24	-0.18	0.29	412%	0	1
Few	0.06	0.24	-0.18	0.29	412%	0	1
Little	1.97	2.35	-0.37	4.32	119%	0	9
Many	0.11	0.40	-0.29	0.52	353%	0	2
Much	0.43	0.81	-0.39	1.24	190%	0	3
One	5.00	3.35	1.65	8.35	67%	0	14
Several	0.00	0.00	0.00	0.00	0%	0	0

Relative	Mean	SD	SD-	SD+	%SD	R-	R+
What	1.26	1.27	-0.01	2.53	101%	0	5
Whatever	0.14	0.43	-0.29	0.57	301%	0	2
Which	0.06	0.24	-0.18	0.29	412%	0	1
Whichever	0.00	0.00	0.00	0.00	0%	0	0
Who	0.31	0.68	-0.36	0.99	215%	0	3
Whoever	0.03	0.17	-0.14	0.20	592%	0	1
Whom	0.00	0.00	0.00	0.00	0%	0	0
Whose	0.06	0.24	-0.18	0.29	412%	0	1

Universal	Mean	SD	SD-	SD+	%SD	R-	R+
All	3.03	2.46	0.57	5.48	81%	0	11
Both	0.11	0.40	-0.29	0.52	353%	0	2
Each	0.06	0.24	-0.18	0.29	412%	0	1
Every	0.23	0.49	-0.26	0.72	214%	0	2
Everybody	0.14	0.43	-0.29	0.57	301%	0	2
Everyone	0.00	0.00	0.00	0.00	0%	0	0
Everything	0.11	0.40	-0.29	0.52	353%	0	2
Everywhere	0.00	0.00	0.00	0.00	0%	0	0

Possessive	Mean	SD	SD-	SD+	%SD	R-	R+
Her	1.89	2.35	-0.46	4.23	125%	0	8
Hers	0.11	0.40	-0.29	0.52	353%	0	2
His	1.46	1.77	-0.31	3.23	122%	0	8
Its	0.06	0.34	-0.28	0.40	592%	0	2
Mine	0.14	0.43	-0.29	0.57	301%	0	2
My	10.37	5.01	5.36	15.38	48%	1	20
Our	1.26	1.58	-0.32	2.84	126%	0	7
Ours	0.03	0.17	-0.14	0.20	592%	0	1
Their	0.54	1.01	-0.47	1.55	186%	0	4
Theirs	0.00	0.00	0.00	0.00	0%	0	0
Your	0.54	0.95	-0.41	1.49	175%	0	4
Yours	0.06	0.24	-0.18	0.29	412%	0	1

Personal	Mean	SD	SD-	SD+	%SD	R-	R+
He	5.14	4.95	0.20	10.09	96%	0	19
Her	1.89	2.35	-0.46	4.23	125%	0	8
Him	1.40	1.29	0.11	2.69	92%	0	5
I	25.51	9.64	15.88	35.15	38%	9	50
It	12.89	7.07	5.81	19.96	55%	3	28
Me	2.86	2.12	0.74	4.97	74%	0	7
She	5.14	6.47	-1.32	11.61	126%	0	26
Them	3.09	3.44	-0.36	6.53	112%	0	18
They	2.71	2.77	-0.06	5.49	102%	0	9
Us	0.66	1.49	-0.84	2.15	227%	0	8
We	8.97	7.68	1.30	16.65	86%	0	27
You	7.20	6.03	1.17	13.23	84%	0	24

Partitive	Mean	SD	SD-	SD+	%SD	R-	R+
Any	0.20	0.47	-0.27	0.67	236%	0	2
Anybody	0.00	0.00	0.00	0.00	0%	0	0
Anyone	0.00	0.00	0.00	0.00	0%	0	0
Anything	0.17	0.45	-0.28	0.62	264%	0	2
Anywhere	0.03	0.17	-0.14	0.20	592%	0	1
Either	0.09	0.37	-0.29	0.46	436%	0	2
Neither	0.03	0.17	-0.14	0.20	592%	0	1
Nobody	0.23	0.65	-0.42	0.87	282%	0	3
None	0.09	0.28	-0.20	0.37	331%	0	1
No one	0.03	0.17	-0.14	0.20	592%	0	1
Nothing	0.40	1.03	-0.63	1.43	259%	0	4
Some	1.71	2.56	-0.85	4.28	149%	0	13
Somebody	0.09	0.28	-0.20	0.37	331%	0	1
Someone	0.17	0.51	-0.34	0.69	300%	0	2
Someplace	0.00	0.00	0.00	0.00	0%	0	0
Something	0.54	0.89	-0.34	1.43	163%	0	3

Word List Summary / 7-Year-Olds
(Conversation: 100 Utterance Samples N=50)

Questions	Mean	SD	SD−	SD+	%SD	R−	R+
How	0.08	0.27	-0.19	0.35	343%	0	1
What	0.44	0.73	-0.29	1.17	167%	0	2
When	0.06	0.24	-0.18	0.30	400%	0	1
Where	0.08	0.27	-0.19	0.35	343%	0	1
Which	0.06	0.42	-0.36	0.48	707%	0	3
Who	0.12	0.39	-0.27	0.51	321%	0	2
Whose	0.00	0.00	0.00	0.00	0%	0	0
Why	0.08	0.44	-0.36	0.52	556%	0	3

Conjunctions	Mean	SD	SD−	SD+	%SD	R−	R+
After	0.30	0.65	-0.35	0.95	216%	0	2
And	30.16	12.89	17.27	43.05	43%	7	76
As	0.48	1.34	-0.86	1.82	280%	0	7
Because	3.40	2.68	0.72	6.08	79%	0	12
But	4.58	3.55	1.03	8.13	77%	0	16
If	1.92	2.44	-0.52	4.36	127%	0	12
Or	1.70	1.80	-0.10	3.50	106%	0	9
Since	0.00	0.00	0.00	0.00	0%	0	0
So	2.26	1.97	0.29	4.23	87%	0	9
Then	5.98	5.07	0.91	11.05	85%	0	21
Until	0.26	0.60	-0.34	0.86	231%	0	2
While	0.10	0.36	-0.26	0.46	364%	0	2

Negatives	Mean	SD	SD−	SD+	%SD	R−	R+
Ain't	0.06	0.24	-0.18	0.30	400%	0	1
Are/n't	0.08	0.27	-0.19	0.35	343%	0	1
Can/n't	1.08	1.10	-0.02	2.18	102%	0	5
Could/n't	0.24	0.62	-0.38	0.86	260%	0	3
Did/n't	0.72	1.14	-0.42	1.86	159%	0	5
Does/n't	0.68	0.79	-0.11	1.47	117%	0	4
Don't	3.80	2.78	1.02	6.58	73%	0	11
Had/n't	0.00	0.00	0.00	0.00	0%	0	0
Has/n't	0.00	0.00	0.00	0.00	0%	0	0
Have/n't	0.10	0.42	-0.32	0.52	416%	0	2
Is/n't	0.14	0.40	-0.26	0.54	289%	0	2
Might/n't	0.00	0.00	0.00	0.00	0%	0	0
Must/n't	0.00	0.00	0.00	0.00	0%	0	0
No	3.30	2.16	1.14	5.46	65%	0	8
Nope	0.22	0.71	-0.49	0.93	322%	0	4
Not	1.84	1.61	0.23	3.45	87%	0	7
Should/n't	0.00	0.00	0.00	0.00	0%	0	0
Uhuh	1.04	1.44	-0.40	2.48	139%	0	5
Was/n't	0.22	0.51	-0.29	0.73	230%	0	2
Were/n't	0.02	0.14	-0.12	0.16	707%	0	1
Won't	0.26	0.60	-0.34	0.86	231%	0	3
Would/n't	0.14	0.40	-0.26	0.54	289%	0	2

Modals	Mean	SD	SD−	SD+	%SD	R−	R+
Can	2.80	2.28	0.52	5.08	81%	0	8
Could	0.68	1.39	-0.71	2.07	205%	0	7
May	0.00	0.00	0.00	0.00	0%	0	0
Might	0.52	1.18	-0.66	1.70	227%	0	7
Must	0.06	0.24	-0.18	0.30	400%	0	1
Shall	0.00	0.00	0.00	0.00	0%	0	0
Should	0.18	0.39	-0.21	0.57	216%	0	1
Will	0.12	0.33	-0.21	0.45	274%	0	1
Would	0.90	1.50	-0.60	2.40	167%	0	8

Pronouns

Reflexive	Mean	SD	SD−	SD+	%SD	R−	R+
Herself	0.02	0.14	-0.12	0.16	707%	0	1
Himself	0.02	0.14	-0.12	0.16	707%	0	1
Itself	0.00	0.00	0.00	0.00	0%	0	0
Myself	0.20	0.45	-0.25	0.65	226%	0	2
Ourselves	0.00	0.00	0.00	0.00	0%	0	0
Themselves	0.00	0.00	0.00	0.00	0%	0	0
Yourself	0.02	0.14	-0.12	0.16	707%	0	1
Yourselves	0.00	0.00	0.00	0.00	0%	0	0

Demonstrative	Mean	SD	SD−	SD+	%SD	R−	R+
That	6.22	3.50	2.72	9.72	56%	2	19
These	0.50	0.95	-0.45	1.45	191%	0	5
This	2.36	2.46	-0.10	4.82	104%	0	10
Those	0.40	0.73	-0.33	1.13	182%	0	3

Quantifying	Mean	SD	SD−	SD+	%SD	R−	R+
Enough	0.08	0.27	-0.19	0.35	343%	0	1
Few	0.02	0.14	-0.12	0.16	707%	0	1
Little	1.84	1.86	-0.02	3.70	101%	0	9
Many	0.18	0.48	-0.30	0.66	268%	0	2
Much	0.58	0.78	-0.20	1.36	135%	0	4
One	4.72	3.00	1.72	7.72	64%	0	14
Several	0.02	0.14	-0.12	0.16	707%	0	1

Relative	Mean	SD	SD−	SD+	%SD	R−	R+
What	0.82	1.04	-0.22	1.86	127%	0	4
Whatever	0.16	0.42	-0.26	0.58	264%	0	2
Which	0.16	0.74	-0.58	0.90	462%	0	5
Whichever	0.02	0.14	-0.12	0.16	707%	0	1
Who	0.28	0.90	-0.62	1.18	323%	0	6
Whoever	0.26	0.78	-0.52	1.04	299%	0	4
Whom	0.00	0.00	0.00	0.00	0%	0	0
Whose	0.00	0.00	0.00	0.00	0%	0	0

Universal	Mean	SD	SD−	SD+	%SD	R−	R+
All	2.78	2.61	0.17	5.39	94%	0	12
Both	0.28	0.67	-0.39	0.95	240%	0	3
Each	0.16	0.62	-0.46	0.78	386%	0	4
Every	0.32	0.71	-0.39	1.03	223%	0	3
Everybody	0.36	0.78	-0.42	1.14	216%	0	3
Everyone	0.14	0.64	-0.50	0.78	457%	0	4
Everything	0.08	0.27	-0.19	0.35	343%	0	1
Everywhere	0.02	0.14	-0.12	0.16	707%	0	1

Possessive	Mean	SD	SD−	SD+	%SD	R−	R+
Her	2.04	3.06	-1.02	5.10	150%	0	15
Hers	0.02	0.14	-0.12	0.16	707%	0	1
His	1.30	1.98	-0.68	3.28	152%	0	10
Its	0.00	0.00	0.00	0.00	0%	0	0
Mine	0.18	0.48	-0.30	0.66	268%	0	2
My	10.76	6.14	4.62	16.90	57%	2	31
Our	1.32	1.90	-0.58	3.22	144%	0	9
Ours	0.00	0.00	0.00	0.00	0%	0	0
Their	0.56	0.93	-0.37	1.49	166%	0	5
Theirs	0.00	0.00	0.00	0.00	0%	0	0
Your	0.84	1.27	-0.43	2.11	151%	0	5
Yours	0.02	0.14	-0.12	0.16	707%	0	1

Personal	Mean	SD	SD−	SD+	%SD	R−	R+
He	6.74	6.37	0.37	13.11	95%	0	27
Her	2.04	3.06	-1.02	5.10	150%	0	15
Him	1.34	1.53	-0.19	2.87	114%	0	6
I	21.92	9.67	12.25	31.59	44%	4	46
It	11.76	6.22	5.54	17.98	53%	2	26
Me	2.94	2.54	0.40	5.48	86%	0	14
She	5.76	6.97	-1.21	12.73	121%	0	29
Them	2.74	2.36	0.38	5.10	86%	0	10
They	4.86	3.03	1.83	7.89	62%	0	13
Us	0.64	1.16	-0.52	1.80	181%	0	6
We	9.72	6.90	2.82	16.62	71%	0	35
You	10.24	9.34	0.90	19.58	91%	0	31

Partitive	Mean	SD	SD−	SD+	%SD	R−	R+
Any	0.30	0.65	-0.35	0.95	216%	0	3
Anybody	0.02	0.14	-0.12	0.16	707%	0	1
Anyone	0.02	0.14	-0.12	0.16	707%	0	1
Anything	0.22	0.51	-0.29	0.73	230%	0	2
Anywhere	0.02	0.14	-0.12	0.16	707%	0	1
Either	0.12	0.39	-0.27	0.51	321%	0	2
Neither	0.02	0.14	-0.12	0.16	707%	0	1
Nobody	0.14	0.40	-0.26	0.54	289%	0	2
None	0.00	0.00	0.00	0.00	0%	0	0
No one	0.10	0.46	-0.36	0.56	463%	0	3
Nothing	0.08	0.40	-0.32	0.48	495%	0	2
Some	1.70	1.54	0.16	3.24	91%	0	8
Somebody	0.42	1.05	-0.63	1.47	250%	0	6
Someone	0.36	0.92	-0.56	1.28	256%	0	4
Someplace	0.04	0.20	-0.16	0.24	495%	0	1
Something	0.66	0.80	-0.14	1.46	121%	0	3

Word List Summary / 9-Year-Olds

(Conversation: 100 Utterance Samples N=27)

Questions

	Mean	SD	SD–	SD+	%SD	R–	R+
How	0.11	0.32	-0.21	0.43	288%	0	1
What	0.37	0.79	-0.42	1.16	214%	0	3
When	0.00	0.00	0.00	0.00	0%	0	0
Where	0.11	0.32	-0.21	0.43	288%	0	1
Which	0.00	0.00	0.00	0.00	0%	0	0
Who	0.00	0.00	0.00	0.00	0%	0	0
Whose	0.00	0.00	0.00	0.00	0%	0	0
Why	0.07	0.38	-0.31	0.46	520%	0	2

Conjunctions

	Mean	SD	SD–	SD+	%SD	R–	R+
After	0.74	0.94	-0.20	1.69	127%	0	3
And	34.85	12.09	22.77	46.94	35%	12	56
As	0.52	1.05	-0.53	1.57	203%	0	4
Because	3.52	3.70	-0.19	7.22	105%	0	14
But	3.41	2.56	0.85	5.97	75%	0	10
If	1.74	1.53	0.21	3.27	88%	0	7
Or	3.22	3.08	0.14	6.30	96%	0	13
Since	0.22	0.42	-0.20	0.65	191%	0	1
So	3.59	3.17	0.43	6.76	88%	0	13
Then	9.07	8.00	1.07	17.07	88%	1	30
Until	0.26	0.53	-0.27	0.78	203%	0	2
While	0.15	0.46	-0.31	0.60	308%	0	2

Negatives

	Mean	SD	SD–	SD+	%SD	R–	R+
Ain't	0.04	0.19	-0.16	0.23	520%	0	1
Are/n't	0.04	0.19	-0.16	0.23	520%	0	1
Can/'t	0.48	0.80	-0.32	1.28	167%	0	3
Could/n't	0.11	0.32	-0.21	0.43	288%	0	1
Did/n't	0.85	1.23	-0.38	2.08	145%	0	4
Does/n't	0.74	1.23	-0.49	1.97	166%	0	4
Don't	2.85	2.85	0.00	5.70	100%	0	11
Had/n't	0.00	0.00	0.00	0.00	0%	0	0
Has/n't	0.07	0.27	-0.19	0.34	360%	0	1
Have/n't	0.11	0.32	-0.21	0.43	288%	0	1
Is/n't	0.11	0.32	-0.21	0.43	288%	0	1
Might/n't	0.00	0.00	0.00	0.00	0%	0	0
Must/n't	0.00	0.00	0.00	0.00	0%	0	0
No	2.70	2.23	0.47	4.94	83%	0	9
Nope	0.07	0.27	-0.19	0.34	360%	0	1
Not	1.85	1.99	-0.14	3.85	108%	0	8
Should/n't	0.00	0.00	0.00	0.00	0%	0	0
Uhuh	0.74	1.23	-0.49	1.97	166%	0	4
Was/n't	0.30	0.54	-0.25	0.84	183%	0	2
Were/n't	0.04	0.19	-0.16	0.23	520%	0	1
Won't	0.07	0.27	-0.19	0.34	360%	0	1
Would/n't	0.07	0.27	-0.19	0.34	360%	0	1

Modals

	Mean	SD	SD–	SD+	%SD	R–	R+
Can	2.26	1.97	0.29	4.23	87%	0	8
Could	0.33	0.68	-0.35	1.01	204%	0	2
May	0.00	0.00	0.00	0.00	0%	0	0
Might	0.30	0.54	-0.25	0.84	183%	0	2
Must	0.04	0.19	-0.16	0.23	520%	0	1
Shall	0.00	0.00	0.00	0.00	0%	0	0
Should	0.07	0.27	-0.19	0.34	360%	0	1
Will	0.37	0.88	-0.51	1.25	239%	0	4
Would	0.74	1.06	-0.32	1.80	143%	0	3

Pronouns

Reflexive

	Mean	SD	SD–	SD+	%SD	R–	R+
Herself	0.04	0.19	-0.16	0.23	520%	0	1
Himself	0.00	0.00	0.00	0.00	0%	0	0
Itself	0.00	0.00	0.00	0.00	0%	0	0
Myself	0.15	0.36	-0.21	0.51	244%	0	1
Ourselves	0.04	0.19	-0.16	0.23	520%	0	1
Themselves	0.00	0.00	0.00	0.00	0%	0	0
Yourself	0.04	0.19	-0.16	0.23	520%	0	1
Yourselves	0.00	0.00	0.00	0.00	0%	0	0

Demonstrative

	Mean	SD	SD–	SD+	%SD	R–	R+
That	8.41	4.13	4.27	12.54	49%	2	23
These	0.37	0.69	-0.32	1.06	186%	0	3
This	2.89	3.36	-0.47	6.24	116%	0	16
Those	0.52	0.89	-0.37	1.41	172%	0	3

Quantifying

	Mean	SD	SD–	SD+	%SD	R–	R+
Enough	0.00	0.00	0.00	0.00	0%	0	0
Few	0.11	0.32	-0.21	0.43	288%	0	1
Little	1.37	1.28	0.09	2.65	93%	0	4
Many	0.19	0.48	-0.30	0.67	261%	0	2
Much	0.56	1.15	-0.60	1.71	208%	0	5
One	4.44	3.25	1.19	7.69	73%	0	14
Several	0.00	0.00	0.00	0.00	0%	0	0

Relative

	Mean	SD	SD–	SD+	%SD	R–	R+
What	1.26	1.46	-0.20	2.72	116%	0	7
Whatever	0.04	0.19	-0.16	0.23	520%	0	1
Which	0.15	0.36	-0.21	0.51	244%	0	1
Whichever	0.00	0.00	0.00	0.00	0%	0	0
Who	0.26	0.66	-0.40	0.92	253%	0	2
Whoever	0.00	0.00	0.00	0.00	0%	0	0
Whom	0.00	0.00	0.00	0.00	0%	0	0
Whose	0.00	0.00	0.00	0.00	0%	0	0

Universal

	Mean	SD	SD–	SD+	%SD	R–	R+
All	2.26	1.56	0.70	3.82	69%	0	7
Both	0.37	0.56	-0.19	0.94	153%	0	2
Each	0.11	0.32	-0.21	0.43	288%	0	1
Every	0.30	0.61	-0.31	0.90	205%	0	2
Everybody	0.19	0.62	-0.44	0.81	336%	0	3
Everyone	0.04	0.19	-0.16	0.23	520%	0	1
Everything	0.26	0.53	-0.27	0.78	203%	0	2
Everywhere	0.00	0.00	0.00	0.00	0%	0	0

Possessive

	Mean	SD	SD–	SD+	%SD	R–	R+
Her	1.74	2.51	-0.76	4.25	144%	0	10
Hers	0.00	0.00	0.00	0.00	0%	0	0
His	0.78	1.09	-0.31	1.86	140%	0	3
Its	0.00	0.00	0.00	0.00	0%	0	0
Mine	0.11	0.32	-0.21	0.43	288%	0	1
My	9.81	5.05	4.76	14.87	51%	1	21
Our	2.78	2.34	0.44	5.12	84%	0	9
Ours	0.00	0.00	0.00	0.00	0%	0	0
Their	0.37	0.69	-0.32	1.06	186%	0	3
Theirs	0.00	0.00	0.00	0.00	0%	0	0
Your	0.56	1.42	-0.87	1.98	256%	0	5
Yours	0.00	0.00	0.00	0.00	0%	0	0

Personal

	Mean	SD	SD–	SD+	%SD	R–	R+
He	4.22	3.45	0.78	7.67	82%	0	12
Her	1.74	2.51	-0.76	4.25	144%	0	10
Him	0.78	1.28	-0.50	2.06	165%	0	5
I	24.19	12.10	12.09	36.28	50%	6	49
It	13.26	6.67	6.59	19.92	50%	3	29
Me	1.89	1.67	0.22	3.56	89%	0	7
She	4.93	4.91	0.01	9.84	100%	0	15
Them	2.26	2.05	0.21	4.31	91%	0	10
They	4.26	3.83	0.43	8.09	90%	0	17
Us	0.67	1.00	-0.33	1.67	150%	0	4
We	19.15	10.18	8.97	29.33	53%	4	45
You	7.70	6.13	1.58	13.83	80%	0	20

Partitive

	Mean	SD	SD–	SD+	%SD	R–	R+
Any	0.48	0.85	-0.37	1.33	176%	0	4
Anybody	0.07	0.27	-0.19	0.34	360%	0	1
Anyone	0.00	0.00	0.00	0.00	0%	0	0
Anything	0.44	0.75	-0.31	1.20	169%	0	3
Anywhere	0.00	0.00	0.00	0.00	0%	0	0
Either	0.37	0.74	-0.37	1.11	200%	0	3
Neither	0.00	0.00	0.00	0.00	0%	0	0
Nobody	0.07	0.27	-0.19	0.34	360%	0	1
None	0.00	0.00	0.00	0.00	0%	0	0
No one	0.19	0.79	-0.60	0.97	425%	0	4
Nothing	0.07	0.27	-0.19	0.34	360%	0	1
Some	1.41	2.04	-0.64	3.45	145%	0	10
Somebody	0.11	0.32	-0.21	0.43	288%	0	1
Someone	0.00	0.00	0.00	0.00	0%	0	0
Someplace	0.00	0.00	0.00	0.00	0%	0	0
Something	1.44	1.09	0.36	2.53	75%	0	4

Word List Summary / 11-Year-Olds
(Conversation: 100 Utterance Samples N=27)

Questions

	Mean	SD	SD–	SD+	%SD	R–	R+
How	0.04	0.19	-0.16	0.23	520%	0	1
What	0.22	0.42	-0.20	0.65	191%	0	1
When	0.04	0.19	-0.16	0.23	520%	0	1
Where	0.07	0.27	-0.19	0.34	360%	0	1
Which	0.04	0.19	-0.16	0.23	520%	0	1
Who	0.00	0.00	0.00	0.00	0%	0	0
Whose	0.00	0.00	0.00	0.00	0%	0	0
Why	0.00	0.00	0.00	0.00	0%	0	0

Conjunctions

	Mean	SD	SD–	SD+	%SD	R–	R+
After	0.93	1.30	-0.37	2.22	140%	0	6
And	39.30	16.45	22.85	55.74	42%	9	72
As	0.44	0.85	-0.40	1.29	191%	0	3
Because	5.26	4.82	0.44	10.08	92%	0	19
But	5.56	3.83	1.73	9.38	69%	0	18
If	1.89	1.83	0.06	3.71	97%	0	6
Or	4.41	4.60	-0.19	9.01	104%	0	23
Since	0.56	1.09	-0.53	1.64	195%	0	4
So	5.11	4.23	0.88	9.34	83%	0	18
Then	9.63	6.97	2.66	16.60	72%	0	20
Until	0.74	1.68	-0.94	2.42	226%	0	8
While	0.44	0.75	-0.31	1.20	169%	0	2

Negatives

	Mean	SD	SD–	SD+	%SD	R–	R+
Ain't	0.04	0.19	-0.16	0.23	520%	0	1
Are/n't	0.15	0.36	-0.21	0.51	244%	0	1
Can/'t	0.70	0.99	-0.29	1.70	141%	0	4
Could/n't	0.19	0.48	-0.30	0.67	261%	0	2
Did/n't	1.00	1.24	-0.24	2.24	124%	0	5
Does/n't	0.37	0.56	-0.19	0.94	153%	0	2
Don't	3.93	2.64	1.28	6.57	67%	0	12
Had/n't	0.00	0.00	0.00	0.00	0%	0	0
Has/n't	0.00	0.00	0.00	0.00	0%	0	0
Have/n't	0.22	0.42	-0.20	0.65	191%	0	1
Is/n't	0.07	0.27	-0.19	0.34	360%	0	1
Might/n't	0.00	0.00	0.00	0.00	0%	0	0
Must/n't	0.00	0.00	0.00	0.00	0%	0	0
No	4.56	2.94	1.62	7.50	65%	0	11
Nope	0.07	0.27	-0.19	0.34	360%	0	1
Not	1.93	1.71	0.22	3.63	89%	0	6
Should/n't	0.00	0.00	0.00	0.00	0%	0	0
Uhuh	0.26	0.53	-0.27	0.78	203%	0	2
Was/n't	0.30	0.54	-0.25	0.84	183%	0	2
Were/n't	0.00	0.00	0.00	0.00	0%	0	0
Won't	0.07	0.38	-0.31	0.46	520%	0	2
Would/n't	0.19	0.40	-0.21	0.58	214%	0	1

Modals

	Mean	SD	SD–	SD+	%SD	R–	R+
Can	2.07	1.86	0.22	3.93	90%	0	5
Could	0.44	0.75	-0.31	1.20	169%	0	2
May	0.15	0.46	-0.31	0.60	308%	0	2
Might	0.48	0.85	-0.37	1.33	176%	0	3
Must	0.00	0.00	0.00	0.00	0%	0	0
Shall	0.00	0.00	0.00	0.00	0%	0	0
Should	0.00	0.00	0.00	0.00	0%	0	0
Will	0.22	0.51	-0.28	0.73	228%	0	2
Would	0.63	1.01	-0.38	1.64	160%	0	4

Pronouns

Reflexive

	Mean	SD	SD–	SD+	%SD	R–	R+
Herself	0.04	0.19	-0.16	0.23	520%	0	1
Himself	0.00	0.00	0.00	0.00	0%	0	0
Itself	0.00	0.00	0.00	0.00	0%	0	0
Myself	0.07	0.27	-0.19	0.34	360%	0	1
Ourselves	0.00	0.00	0.00	0.00	0%	0	0
Themselves	0.00	0.00	0.00	0.00	0%	0	0
Yourself	0.00	0.00	0.00	0.00	0%	0	0
Yourselves	0.00	0.00	0.00	0.00	0%	0	0

Demonstrative

	Mean	SD	SD–	SD+	%SD	R–	R+
That	8.30	4.50	3.79	12.80	54%	2	21
These	0.11	0.42	-0.31	0.53	381%	0	2
This	2.41	2.79	-0.38	5.20	116%	0	11
Those	0.48	0.80	-0.32	1.28	167%	0	3

Quantifying

	Mean	SD	SD–	SD+	%SD	R–	R+
Enough	0.19	0.48	-0.30	0.67	261%	0	2
Few	0.37	0.69	-0.32	1.06	186%	0	2
Little	1.15	1.20	-0.05	2.35	104%	0	4
Many	0.30	0.47	-0.17	0.76	157%	0	1
Much	1.04	1.22	-0.19	2.26	118%	0	4
One	5.74	4.63	1.11	10.37	81%	0	18
Several	0.00	0.00	0.00	0.00	0%	0	0

Relative

	Mean	SD	SD–	SD+	%SD	R–	R+
What	1.11	1.28	-0.17	2.39	115%	0	5
Whatever	0.30	0.61	-0.31	0.90	205%	0	2
Which	0.33	0.92	-0.59	1.25	276%	0	4
Whichever	0.00	0.00	0.00	0.00	0%	0	0
Who	0.33	0.68	-0.35	1.01	204%	0	2
Whoever	0.04	0.19	-0.16	0.23	520%	0	1
Whom	0.00	0.00	0.00	0.00	0%	0	0
Whose	0.00	0.00	0.00	0.00	0%	0	0

Universal

	Mean	SD	SD–	SD+	%SD	R–	R+
All	3.04	2.05	0.99	5.08	67%	0	9
Both	0.44	0.75	-0.31	1.20	169%	0	2
Each	0.37	0.79	-0.42	1.16	214%	0	3
Every	0.93	1.24	-0.31	2.16	134%	0	5
Everybody	0.33	0.73	-0.40	1.07	220%	0	3
Everyone	0.30	0.61	-0.31	0.90	205%	0	2
Everything	0.52	0.80	-0.28	1.32	155%	0	3
Everywhere	0.00	0.00	0.00	0.00	0%	0	0

Possessive

	Mean	SD	SD–	SD+	%SD	R–	R+
Her	1.67	2.29	-0.62	3.95	137%	0	8
Hers	0.00	0.00	0.00	0.00	0%	0	0
His	0.96	1.16	-0.20	2.12	120%	0	5
Its	0.00	0.00	0.00	0.00	0%	0	0
Mine	0.11	0.42	-0.31	0.53	381%	0	2
My	17.37	10.21	7.16	27.58	59%	2	42
Our	3.33	2.48	0.85	5.81	74%	0	10
Ours	0.00	0.00	0.00	0.00	0%	0	0
Their	0.56	0.93	-0.38	1.49	168%	0	4
Theirs	0.00	0.00	0.00	0.00	0%	0	0
Your	0.67	1.30	-0.63	1.97	195%	0	4
Yours	0.00	0.00	0.00	0.00	0%	0	0

Personal

	Mean	SD	SD–	SD+	%SD	R–	R+
He	5.48	5.21	0.27	10.70	95%	0	19
Her	1.67	2.29	-0.62	3.95	137%	0	8
Him	0.81	1.14	-0.33	1.96	140%	0	4
I	25.15	11.68	13.47	36.83	46%	10	54
It	11.33	7.59	3.74	18.92	67%	1	35
Me	2.19	1.59	0.59	3.78	73%	0	5
She	4.67	5.59	-0.92	10.26	120%	0	26
Them	2.89	2.64	0.25	5.52	91%	0	10
They	5.89	4.05	1.84	9.94	69%	0	16
Us	1.00	1.54	-0.54	2.54	154%	0	6
We	22.74	9.28	13.46	32.02	41%	8	43
You	6.04	8.09	-2.06	14.13	134%	0	35

Partitive

	Mean	SD	SD–	SD+	%SD	R–	R+
Any	0.30	0.54	-0.25	0.84	183%	0	2
Anybody	0.07	0.27	-0.19	0.34	360%	0	1
Anyone	0.07	0.27	-0.19	0.34	360%	0	1
Anything	0.37	0.74	-0.37	1.11	200%	0	3
Anywhere	0.00	0.00	0.00	0.00	0%	0	0
Either	0.30	0.61	-0.31	0.90	205%	0	2
Neither	0.04	0.19	-0.16	0.23	520%	0	1
Nobody	0.07	0.27	-0.19	0.34	360%	0	1
None	0.07	0.27	-0.19	0.34	360%	0	1
No one	0.04	0.19	-0.16	0.23	520%	0	1
Nothing	0.22	0.51	-0.28	0.73	228%	0	2
Some	1.33	1.73	-0.40	3.07	130%	0	5
Somebody	0.22	0.58	-0.36	0.80	260%	0	2
Someone	0.11	0.32	-0.21	0.43	288%	0	1
Someplace	0.00	0.00	0.00	0.00	0%	0	0
Something	1.56	2.01	-0.45	3.56	129%	0	9

Word List Summary / 13-Year-Olds
(Conversation: 100 Utterance Samples N=27)

Questions	Mean	SD	SD–	SD+	%SD	R–	R+
How	0.00	0.00	0.00	0.00	0%	0	0
What	0.93	1.33	-0.40	2.25	143%	0	5
When	0.11	0.32	-0.21	0.43	288%	0	1
Where	0.11	0.42	-0.31	0.53	381%	0	2
Which	0.04	0.19	-0.16	0.23	520%	0	1
Who	0.00	0.00	0.00	0.00	0%	0	0
Whose	0.00	0.00	0.00	0.00	0%	0	0
Why	0.00	0.00	0.00	0.00	0%	0	0

Conjunctions	Mean	SD	SD–	SD+	%SD	R–	R+
After	1.89	2.62	-0.73	4.51	139%	0	12
And	35.85	13.20	22.65	49.05	37%	17	59
As	0.41	0.75	-0.34	1.15	183%	0	2
Because	3.70	3.26	0.45	6.96	88%	0	13
But	5.96	4.58	1.38	10.54	77%	0	17
If	1.48	1.63	-0.14	3.11	110%	0	6
Or	3.89	3.71	0.17	7.60	96%	0	14
Since	0.15	0.36	-0.21	0.51	244%	0	1
So	4.89	4.28	0.61	9.17	88%	0	17
Then	11.15	5.97	5.18	17.11	54%	0	22
Until	0.48	0.75	-0.27	1.23	156%	0	3
While	0.30	0.54	-0.25	0.84	183%	0	2

Negatives	Mean	SD	SD–	SD+	%SD	R–	R+
Ain't	0.00	0.00	0.00	0.00	0%	0	0
Are/n't	0.04	0.19	-0.16	0.23	520%	0	1
Can't	0.70	0.99	-0.29	1.70	141%	0	3
Could/n't	0.04	0.19	-0.16	0.23	520%	0	1
Did/n't	0.85	1.17	-0.32	2.02	137%	0	5
Does/n't	0.52	0.70	-0.18	1.22	135%	0	2
Don't	4.52	3.13	1.39	7.65	69%	1	15
Had/n't	0.00	0.00	0.00	0.00	0%	0	0
Has/n't	0.00	0.00	0.00	0.00	0%	0	0
Have/n't	0.41	0.57	-0.16	0.98	140%	0	2
Is/n't	0.19	0.48	-0.30	0.67	261%	0	2
Might/n't	0.00	0.00	0.00	0.00	0%	0	0
Must/n't	0.00	0.00	0.00	0.00	0%	0	0
No	4.26	2.77	1.49	7.03	65%	0	9
Nope	0.00	0.00	0.00	0.00	0%	0	0
Not	2.19	1.86	0.32	4.05	85%	0	6
Should/n't	0.00	0.00	0.00	0.00	0%	0	0
Uhuh	0.52	0.94	-0.42	1.45	180%	0	4
Was/n't	0.22	0.51	-0.28	0.73	228%	0	2
Were/n't	0.04	0.19	-0.16	0.23	520%	0	1
Won't	0.26	0.45	-0.19	0.71	172%	0	1
Would/n't	0.04	0.19	-0.16	0.23	520%	0	1

Modals	Mean	SD	SD–	SD+	%SD	R–	R+
Can	2.37	1.92	0.45	4.29	81%	0	6
Could	0.48	0.80	-0.32	1.28	167%	0	3
May	0.04	0.19	-0.16	0.23	520%	0	1
Might	0.44	1.25	-0.81	1.70	281%	0	5
Must	0.00	0.00	0.00	0.00	0%	0	0
Shall	0.00	0.00	0.00	0.00	0%	0	0
Should	0.11	0.42	-0.31	0.53	381%	0	2
Will	0.19	0.40	-0.21	0.58	214%	0	1
Would	0.44	0.80	-0.36	1.25	180%	0	3

Pronouns

Reflexive	Mean	SD	SD–	SD+	%SD	R–	R+
Herself	0.00	0.00	0.00	0.00	0%	0	0
Himself	0.00	0.00	0.00	0.00	0%	0	0
Itself	0.00	0.00	0.00	0.00	0%	0	0
Myself	0.11	0.42	-0.31	0.53	381%	0	2
Ourselves	0.00	0.00	0.00	0.00	0%	0	0
Themselves	0.04	0.19	-0.16	0.23	520%	0	1
Yourself	0.04	0.19	-0.16	0.23	520%	0	1
Yourselves	0.00	0.00	0.00	0.00	0%	0	0

Demonstrative	Mean	SD	SD–	SD+	%SD	R–	R+
That	9.74	5.72	4.02	15.46	59%	1	19
These	0.41	0.89	-0.48	1.30	218%	0	3
This	2.41	2.44	-0.03	4.85	101%	0	10
Those	0.44	0.80	-0.36	1.25	180%	0	3

Quantifying	Mean	SD	SD–	SD+	%SD	R–	R+
Enough	0.00	0.00	0.00	0.00	0%	0	0
Few	0.22	0.51	-0.28	0.73	228%	0	2
Little	1.59	1.87	-0.27	3.46	117%	0	9
Many	0.04	0.19	-0.16	0.23	520%	0	1
Much	0.78	1.05	-0.27	1.83	135%	0	3
One	1.85	1.46	0.39	3.31	79%	0	5
Several	0.00	0.00	0.00	0.00	0%	0	0

Relative	Mean	SD	SD–	SD+	%SD	R–	R+
What	1.67	1.80	-0.13	3.46	108%	0	7
Whatever	0.37	0.74	-0.37	1.11	200%	0	3
Which	0.56	1.01	-0.46	1.57	182%	0	4
Whichever	0.00	0.00	0.00	0.00	0%	0	0
Who	0.19	0.48	-0.30	0.67	261%	0	2
Whoever	0.00	0.00	0.00	0.00	0%	0	0
Whom	0.00	0.00	0.00	0.00	0%	0	0
Whose	0.00	0.00	0.00	0.00	0%	0	0

Universal	Mean	SD	SD–	SD+	%SD	R–	R+
All	3.22	2.91	0.31	6.14	90%	0	11
Both	0.33	0.55	-0.22	0.89	166%	0	2
Each	0.22	0.58	-0.36	0.80	260%	0	2
Every	0.52	0.89	-0.37	1.41	172%	0	3
Everybody	0.15	0.36	-0.21	0.51	244%	0	1
Everyone	0.07	0.38	-0.31	0.46	520%	0	2
Everything	1.00	1.57	-0.57	2.57	157%	0	6
Everywhere	0.00	0.00	0.00	0.00	0%	0	0

Possessive	Mean	SD	SD–	SD+	%SD	R–	R+
Her	1.52	2.08	-0.56	3.60	137%	0	7
Hers	0.04	0.19	-0.16	0.23	520%	0	1
His	0.67	0.92	-0.25	1.59	138%	0	3
Its	0.00	0.00	0.00	0.00	0%	0	0
Mine	0.07	0.27	-0.19	0.34	360%	0	1
My	9.48	4.81	4.67	14.29	51%	1	24
Our	1.07	1.38	-0.31	2.46	129%	0	5
Ours	0.07	0.27	-0.19	0.34	360%	0	1
Their	0.59	1.12	-0.53	1.71	189%	0	5
Theirs	0.00	0.00	0.00	0.00	0%	0	0
Your	0.44	0.75	-0.31	1.20	169%	0	3
Yours	0.00	0.00	0.00	0.00	0%	0	0

Personal	Mean	SD	SD–	SD+	%SD	R–	R+
He	4.15	3.61	0.54	7.76	87%	0	12
Her	1.52	2.08	-0.56	3.60	137%	0	7
Him	0.89	1.53	-0.64	2.42	172%	0	7
I	33.26	15.21	18.05	48.47	46%	6	68
It	15.74	6.48	9.26	22.22	41%	5	31
Me	2.15	1.83	0.31	3.98	85%	0	5
She	3.74	3.22	0.52	6.96	86%	0	10
Them	2.52	2.46	0.06	4.97	97%	0	9
They	4.48	4.26	0.22	8.75	95%	0	15
Us	1.04	1.13	-0.09	2.16	109%	0	3
We	15.44	7.29	8.15	22.74	47%	2	33
You	8.52	7.37	1.15	15.88	86%	0	28

Partitive	Mean	SD	SD–	SD+	%SD	R–	R+
Any	0.44	0.80	-0.36	1.25	180%	0	3
Anybody	0.04	0.19	-0.16	0.23	520%	0	1
Anyone	0.04	0.19	-0.16	0.23	520%	0	1
Anything	0.30	0.61	-0.31	0.90	205%	0	2
Anywhere	0.04	0.19	-0.16	0.23	520%	0	1
Either	0.41	0.64	-0.23	1.04	156%	0	2
Neither	0.04	0.19	-0.16	0.23	520%	0	1
Nobody	0.07	0.27	-0.19	0.34	360%	0	1
None	0.00	0.00	0.00	0.00	0%	0	0
No one	0.00	0.00	0.00	0.00	0%	0	0
Nothing	0.26	0.66	-0.40	0.92	253%	0	3
Some	0.89	1.37	-0.48	2.26	154%	0	6
Somebody	0.11	0.32	-0.21	0.43	288%	0	1
Someone	0.04	0.19	-0.16	0.23	520%	0	1
Someplace	0.07	0.38	-0.31	0.46	520%	0	2
Something	1.59	2.44	-0.85	4.03	153%	0	11

Word List Summary / 3-Year-Olds

(Narration: 100 Utterance Samples N=42)

Questions

	Mean	SD	SD–	SD+	%SD	R–	R+
How	0.31	0.75	-0.44	1.06	242%	0	4
What	3.60	3.84	-0.25	7.44	107%	0	14
When	0.05	0.22	-0.17	0.26	453%	0	1
Where	0.76	1.10	-0.34	1.86	144%	0	4
Which	0.10	0.48	-0.39	0.58	509%	0	3
Who	0.38	0.94	-0.55	1.32	246%	0	5
Whose	0.00	0.00	0.00	0.00	0%	0	0
Why	1.07	1.60	-0.53	2.67	149%	0	7

Conjunctions

	Mean	SD	SD–	SD+	%SD	R–	R+
After	0.17	0.44	-0.27	0.60	262%	0	2
And	15.02	12.24	2.78	27.27	81%	1	46
As	0.00	0.00	0.00	0.00	0%	0	0
Because	1.00	1.62	-0.62	2.62	162%	0	8
But	1.12	2.15	-1.04	3.27	193%	0	10
If	0.24	0.53	-0.29	0.77	224%	0	2
Or	0.14	0.47	-0.33	0.62	331%	0	2
Since	0.00	0.00	0.00	0.00	0%	0	0
So	0.62	1.48	-0.86	2.10	239%	0	8
Then	4.62	6.33	-1.71	10.95	137%	0	30
Until	0.05	0.31	-0.26	0.36	648%	0	2
While	0.05	0.22	-0.17	0.26	453%	0	1

Negatives

	Mean	SD	SD–	SD+	%SD	R–	R+
Ain't	0.00	0.00	0.00	0.00	0%	0	0
Are/n't	0.00	0.00	0.00	0.00	0%	0	0
Can/'t	0.50	1.04	-0.54	1.54	208%	0	6
Could/n't	0.12	0.50	-0.38	0.62	423%	0	3
Did/n't	0.62	1.01	-0.39	1.63	163%	0	4
Does/n't	0.21	0.47	-0.26	0.68	220%	0	2
Don't	4.69	6.28	-1.59	10.97	134%	0	27
Had/n't	0.00	0.00	0.00	0.00	0%	0	0
Has/n't	0.00	0.00	0.00	0.00	0%	0	0
Have/n't	0.00	0.00	0.00	0.00	0%	0	0
Is/n't	0.05	0.22	-0.17	0.26	453%	0	1
Might/n't	0.00	0.00	0.00	0.00	0%	0	0
Must/n't	0.00	0.00	0.00	0.00	0%	0	0
No	3.50	3.24	0.26	6.74	93%	0	15
Nope	0.24	0.48	-0.25	0.72	203%	0	2
Not	0.71	0.89	-0.18	1.61	125%	0	3
Should/n't	0.12	0.63	-0.51	0.75	531%	0	4
Uhuh	0.57	2.03	-1.45	2.60	355%	0	13
Was/n't	0.02	0.15	-0.13	0.18	648%	0	1
Were/n't	0.00	0.00	0.00	0.00	0%	0	0
Won't	0.21	0.56	-0.35	0.78	263%	0	3
Would/n't	0.00	0.00	0.00	0.00	0%	0	0

Modals

	Mean	SD	SD–	SD+	%SD	R–	R+
Can	1.17	1.21	-0.04	2.37	104%	0	6
Could	0.19	0.80	-0.61	0.99	422%	0	5
May	0.02	0.15	-0.13	0.18	648%	0	1
Might	0.10	0.30	-0.20	0.39	312%	0	1
Must	0.02	0.15	-0.13	0.18	648%	0	1
Shall	0.00	0.00	0.00	0.00	0%	0	0
Should	0.31	0.84	-0.53	1.15	272%	0	4
Will	0.52	1.11	-0.59	1.63	212%	0	6
Would	0.10	0.37	-0.27	0.47	389%	0	2

Pronouns

Reflexive

	Mean	SD	SD–	SD+	%SD	R–	R+
Herself	0.02	0.15	-0.13	0.18	648%	0	1
Himself	0.00	0.00	0.00	0.00	0%	0	0
Itself	0.00	0.00	0.00	0.00	0%	0	0
Myself	0.10	0.37	-0.27	0.47	389%	0	2
Ourselves	0.00	0.00	0.00	0.00	0%	0	0
Themselves	0.00	0.00	0.00	0.00	0%	0	0
Yourself	0.02	0.15	-0.13	0.18	648%	0	1
Yourselves	0.00	0.00	0.00	0.00	0%	0	0

Demonstrative

	Mean	SD	SD–	SD+	%SD	R–	R+
That	7.29	4.15	3.13	11.44	57%	1	21
These	0.69	1.26	-0.57	1.95	182%	0	6
This	6.90	5.92	0.99	12.82	86%	0	29
Those	0.50	0.97	-0.47	1.47	194%	0	4

Quantifying

	Mean	SD	SD–	SD+	%SD	R–	R+
Enough	0.00	0.00	0.00	0.00	0%	0	0
Few	0.00	0.00	0.00	0.00	0%	0	0
Little	1.81	2.46	-0.65	4.27	136%	0	12
Many	0.02	0.15	-0.13	0.18	648%	0	1
Much	0.02	0.15	-0.13	0.18	648%	0	1
One	4.74	3.86	0.87	8.60	82%	0	17
Several	0.00	0.00	0.00	0.00	0%	0	0

Relative

	Mean	SD	SD–	SD+	%SD	R–	R+
What	0.67	1.03	-0.36	1.69	154%	0	3
Whatever	0.00	0.00	0.00	0.00	0%	0	0
Which	0.21	0.90	-0.68	1.11	419%	0	5
Whichever	0.00	0.00	0.00	0.00	0%	0	0
Who	0.19	0.63	-0.44	0.82	333%	0	3
Whoever	0.00	0.00	0.00	0.00	0%	0	0
Whom	0.00	0.00	0.00	0.00	0%	0	0
Whose	0.00	0.00	0.00	0.00	0%	0	0

Universal

	Mean	SD	SD–	SD+	%SD	R–	R+
All	1.93	2.35	-0.42	4.28	122%	0	9
Both	0.00	0.00	0.00	0.00	0%	0	0
Each	0.05	0.31	-0.26	0.36	648%	0	2
Every	0.00	0.00	0.00	0.00	0%	0	0
Everybody	0.02	0.15	-0.13	0.18	648%	0	1
Everyone	0.02	0.15	-0.13	0.18	648%	0	1
Everything	0.02	0.15	-0.13	0.18	648%	0	1
Everywhere	0.00	0.00	0.00	0.00	0%	0	0

Possessive

	Mean	SD	SD–	SD+	%SD	R–	R+
Her	2.67	3.43	-0.76	6.09	128%	0	20
Hers	0.05	0.22	-0.17	0.26	453%	0	1
His	1.88	3.10	-1.22	4.98	165%	0	14
Its	0.00	0.00	0.00	0.00	0%	0	0
Mine	0.14	0.35	-0.21	0.50	248%	0	1
My	3.74	3.61	0.13	7.35	97%	0	13
Our	0.14	0.35	-0.21	0.50	248%	0	1
Ours	0.00	0.00	0.00	0.00	0%	0	0
Their	0.48	0.97	-0.49	1.44	203%	0	5
Theirs	0.05	0.31	-0.26	0.36	648%	0	2
Your	0.29	0.77	-0.49	1.06	271%	0	4
Yours	0.05	0.22	-0.17	0.26	453%	0	1

Personal

	Mean	SD	SD–	SD+	%SD	R–	R+
He	7.55	7.10	0.44	14.65	94%	0	31
Her	2.67	3.43	-0.76	6.09	128%	0	20
Him	1.52	1.88	-0.35	3.40	123%	0	7
I	12.07	8.92	3.15	20.99	74%	0	40
It	6.43	4.93	1.49	11.36	77%	0	20
Me	1.00	1.51	-0.51	2.51	151%	0	6
She	6.95	7.34	-0.38	14.29	106%	0	25
Them	0.83	1.43	-0.60	2.26	172%	0	8
They	4.19	3.83	0.36	8.02	91%	0	15
Us	0.00	0.00	0.00	0.00	0%	0	0
We	0.90	1.49	-0.59	2.40	165%	0	7
You	2.74	2.39	0.35	5.13	87%	0	10

Partitive

	Mean	SD	SD–	SD+	%SD	R–	R+
Any	0.12	0.33	-0.21	0.45	275%	0	1
Anybody	0.02	0.15	-0.13	0.18	648%	0	1
Anyone	0.00	0.00	0.00	0.00	0%	0	0
Anything	0.02	0.15	-0.13	0.18	648%	0	1
Anywhere	0.00	0.00	0.00	0.00	0%	0	0
Either	0.00	0.00	0.00	0.00	0%	0	0
Neither	0.00	0.00	0.00	0.00	0%	0	0
Nobody	0.07	0.26	-0.19	0.33	365%	0	1
None	0.02	0.15	-0.13	0.18	648%	0	1
No one	0.00	0.00	0.00	0.00	0%	0	0
Nothing	0.36	1.74	-1.38	2.09	486%	0	11
Some	1.10	1.25	-0.15	2.34	114%	0	5
Somebody	0.62	1.40	-0.78	2.02	226%	0	7
Someone	0.67	2.00	-1.33	2.66	299%	0	9
Someplace	0.00	0.00	0.00	0.00	0%	0	0
Something	0.33	0.90	-0.57	1.24	271%	0	5

Word List Summary / 4-Year-Olds

(Narration: 100 Utterance Samples N=30)

Questions

	Mean	SD	SD–	SD+	%SD	R–	R+
How	0.17	0.46	-0.29	0.63	277%	0	2
What	1.97	2.09	-0.13	4.06	106%	0	7
When	0.17	0.38	-0.21	0.55	227%	0	1
Where	0.13	0.35	-0.21	0.48	259%	0	1
Which	0.00	0.00	0.00	0.00	0%	0	0
Who	0.17	0.38	-0.21	0.55	227%	0	1
Whose	0.00	0.00	0.00	0.00	0%	0	0
Why	0.30	0.65	-0.35	0.95	217%	0	2

Conjunctions

	Mean	SD	SD–	SD+	%SD	R–	R+
After	0.37	0.67	-0.30	1.04	182%	0	2
And	28.00	14.15	13.85	42.15	51%	4	58
As	0.07	0.37	-0.30	0.43	548%	0	2
Because	2.03	2.33	-0.29	4.36	114%	0	11
But	4.33	4.10	0.23	8.44	95%	0	19
If	0.23	0.63	-0.39	0.86	268%	0	3
Or	0.27	0.52	-0.25	0.79	195%	0	2
Since	0.00	0.00	0.00	0.00	0%	0	0
So	1.23	2.22	-0.99	3.46	180%	0	10
Then	10.40	9.38	1.02	19.78	90%	0	33
Until	0.13	0.43	-0.30	0.57	326%	0	2
While	0.03	0.18	-0.15	0.22	548%	0	1

Negatives

	Mean	SD	SD–	SD+	%SD	R–	R+
Ain't	0.00	0.00	0.00	0.00	0%	0	0
Are/n't	0.07	0.25	-0.19	0.32	381%	0	1
Can/'t	0.80	1.19	-0.39	1.99	148%	0	4
Could/n't	0.37	0.61	-0.25	0.98	168%	0	2
Did/n't	1.13	1.63	-0.50	2.77	144%	0	6
Does/n't	0.37	0.61	-0.25	0.98	168%	0	2
Don't	4.97	3.68	1.29	8.65	74%	0	13
Had/n't	0.00	0.00	0.00	0.00	0%	0	0
Has/n't	0.00	0.00	0.00	0.00	0%	0	0
Have/n't	0.03	0.18	-0.15	0.22	548%	0	1
Is/n't	0.07	0.25	-0.19	0.32	381%	0	1
Might/n't	0.00	0.00	0.00	0.00	0%	0	0
Must/n't	0.00	0.00	0.00	0.00	0%	0	0
No	5.17	3.83	1.33	9.00	74%	0	18
Nope	0.20	0.48	-0.28	0.68	242%	0	2
Not	1.17	1.02	0.15	2.19	87%	0	3
Should/n't	0.00	0.00	0.00	0.00	0%	0	0
Uhuh	0.83	1.64	-0.81	2.48	197%	0	7
Was/n't	0.27	0.58	-0.32	0.85	219%	0	2
Were/n't	0.07	0.25	-0.19	0.32	381%	0	1
Won't	0.17	0.65	-0.48	0.81	389%	0	3
Would/n't	0.00	0.00	0.00	0.00	0%	0	0

Modals

	Mean	SD	SD–	SD+	%SD	R–	R+
Can	2.30	2.07	0.23	4.37	90%	0	9
Could	0.87	1.17	-0.30	2.03	135%	0	5
May	0.03	0.18	-0.15	0.22	548%	0	1
Might	0.07	0.25	-0.19	0.32	381%	0	1
Must	0.00	0.00	0.00	0.00	0%	0	0
Shall	0.00	0.00	0.00	0.00	0%	0	0
Should	0.10	0.31	-0.21	0.41	305%	0	1
Will	0.33	0.84	-0.51	1.18	253%	0	4
Would	0.20	0.48	-0.28	0.68	242%	0	2

Pronouns

Reflexive

	Mean	SD	SD–	SD+	%SD	R–	R+
Herself	0.07	0.25	-0.19	0.32	381%	0	1
Himself	0.00	0.00	0.00	0.00	0%	0	0
Itself	0.00	0.00	0.00	0.00	0%	0	0
Myself	0.00	0.00	0.00	0.00	0%	0	0
Ourselves	0.00	0.00	0.00	0.00	0%	0	0
Themselves	0.00	0.00	0.00	0.00	0%	0	0
Yourself	0.00	0.00	0.00	0.00	0%	0	0
Yourselves	0.00	0.00	0.00	0.00	0%	0	0

Demonstrative

	Mean	SD	SD–	SD+	%SD	R–	R+
That	7.50	3.37	4.13	10.87	45%	2	16
These	0.23	0.57	-0.33	0.80	244%	0	2
This	1.80	1.58	0.22	3.38	88%	0	7
Those	0.60	1.10	-0.50	1.70	184%	0	4

Quantifying

	Mean	SD	SD–	SD+	%SD	R–	R+
Enough	0.03	0.18	-0.15	0.22	548%	0	1
Few	0.07	0.37	-0.30	0.43	548%	0	2
Little	1.97	2.03	-0.06	3.99	103%	0	6
Many	0.13	0.57	-0.44	0.70	429%	0	3
Much	0.23	0.50	-0.27	0.74	216%	0	2
One	4.90	3.90	1.00	8.80	80%	0	18
Several	0.00	0.00	0.00	0.00	0%	0	0

Relative

	Mean	SD	SD–	SD+	%SD	R–	R+
What	0.80	1.10	-0.30	1.90	137%	0	4
Whatever	0.00	0.00	0.00	0.00	0%	0	0
Which	0.07	0.25	-0.19	0.32	381%	0	1
Whichever	0.00	0.00	0.00	0.00	0%	0	0
Who	0.33	0.61	-0.27	0.94	182%	0	2
Whoever	0.00	0.00	0.00	0.00	0%	0	0
Whom	0.00	0.00	0.00	0.00	0%	0	0
Whose	0.00	0.00	0.00	0.00	0%	0	0

Universal

	Mean	SD	SD–	SD+	%SD	R–	R+
All	3.07	3.10	-0.03	6.16	101%	0	10
Both	0.07	0.25	-0.19	0.32	381%	0	1
Each	0.00	0.00	0.00	0.00	0%	0	0
Every	0.13	0.35	-0.21	0.48	259%	0	1
Everybody	0.10	0.31	-0.21	0.41	305%	0	1
Everyone	0.00	0.00	0.00	0.00	0%	0	0
Everything	0.27	0.64	-0.37	0.91	240%	0	2
Everywhere	0.03	0.18	-0.15	0.22	548%	0	1

Possessive

	Mean	SD	SD–	SD+	%SD	R–	R+
Her	2.57	3.18	-0.61	5.75	124%	0	12
Hers	0.00	0.00	0.00	0.00	0%	0	0
His	1.70	2.09	-0.39	3.79	123%	0	8
Its	0.00	0.00	0.00	0.00	0%	0	0
Mine	0.17	0.59	-0.43	0.76	355%	0	3
My	4.00	2.94	1.06	6.94	73%	0	10
Our	0.37	0.96	-0.60	1.33	263%	0	4
Ours	0.00	0.00	0.00	0.00	0%	0	0
Their	1.47	1.66	-0.19	3.12	113%	0	5
Theirs	0.00	0.00	0.00	0.00	0%	0	0
Your	0.30	0.60	-0.30	0.90	199%	0	2
Yours	0.03	0.18	-0.15	0.22	548%	0	1

Personal

	Mean	SD	SD–	SD+	%SD	R–	R+
He	7.73	4.84	2.89	12.58	63%	1	21
Her	2.57	3.18	-0.61	5.75	124%	0	12
Him	1.47	1.96	-0.49	3.43	134%	0	7
I	18.67	8.44	10.23	27.10	45%	4	33
It	10.00	6.82	3.18	16.82	68%	2	31
Me	1.57	1.28	0.29	2.84	82%	0	5
She	8.07	7.99	0.08	16.05	99%	0	25
Them	1.80	2.06	-0.26	3.86	114%	0	7
They	5.20	3.58	1.62	8.78	69%	1	14
Us	0.07	0.25	-0.19	0.32	381%	0	1
We	1.50	1.89	-0.39	3.39	126%	0	7
You	4.90	4.35	0.55	9.25	89%	0	19

Partitive

	Mean	SD	SD–	SD+	%SD	R–	R+
Any	0.47	0.63	-0.16	1.10	135%	0	2
Anybody	0.00	0.00	0.00	0.00	0%	0	0
Anyone	0.07	0.25	-0.19	0.32	381%	0	1
Anything	0.07	0.25	-0.19	0.32	381%	0	1
Anywhere	0.00	0.00	0.00	0.00	0%	0	0
Either	0.13	0.35	-0.21	0.48	259%	0	1
Neither	0.00	0.00	0.00	0.00	0%	0	0
Nobody	0.03	0.18	-0.15	0.22	548%	0	1
None	0.07	0.25	-0.19	0.32	381%	0	1
No one	0.03	0.18	-0.15	0.22	548%	0	1
Nothing	0.13	0.35	-0.21	0.48	259%	0	1
Some	1.67	1.90	-0.23	3.57	114%	0	9
Somebody	0.43	1.04	-0.61	1.47	240%	0	5
Someone	0.87	2.11	-1.25	2.98	244%	0	8
Someplace	0.00	0.00	0.00	0.00	0%	0	0
Something	0.13	0.43	-0.30	0.57	326%	0	2

Word List Summary / 5-Year-Olds
(Narration: 100 Utterance Samples N=28)

Questions	Mean	SD	SD–	SD+	%SD	R–	R+
How	0.25	0.52	-0.27	0.77	207%	0	2
What	2.18	1.98	0.20	4.16	91%	0	7
When	0.04	0.19	-0.15	0.22	529%	0	1
Where	0.32	0.86	-0.54	1.18	268%	0	3
Which	0.00	0.00	0.00	0.00	0%	0	0
Who	0.61	1.57	-0.96	2.18	259%	0	8
Whose	0.00	0.00	0.00	0.00	0%	0	0
Why	0.43	0.84	-0.41	1.26	195%	0	3

Conjunctions	Mean	SD	SD–	SD+	%SD	R–	R+
After	0.25	0.52	-0.27	0.77	207%	0	2
And	32.39	16.16	16.24	48.55	50%	9	68
As	0.07	0.26	-0.19	0.33	367%	0	1
Because	2.18	2.40	-0.23	4.58	110%	0	10
But	3.57	2.43	1.15	6.00	68%	0	9
If	0.86	1.51	-0.65	2.37	176%	0	7
Or	0.68	1.22	-0.54	1.90	180%	0	5
Since	0.00	0.00	0.00	0.00	0%	0	0
So	2.14	2.58	-0.44	4.72	120%	0	10
Then	14.04	11.04	3.00	25.08	79%	2	48
Until	0.11	0.31	-0.21	0.42	294%	0	1
While	0.07	0.26	-0.19	0.33	367%	0	1

Negatives	Mean	SD	SD–	SD+	%SD	R–	R+
Ain't	0.04	0.19	-0.15	0.22	529%	0	1
Are/n't	0.07	0.26	-0.19	0.33	367%	0	1
Can't	1.07	1.49	-0.42	2.56	139%	0	6
Could/n't	0.54	0.88	-0.35	1.42	164%	0	3
Did/n't	1.00	1.02	-0.02	2.02	102%	0	3
Does/n't	0.32	0.82	-0.50	1.14	255%	0	3
Don't	6.18	4.31	1.87	10.49	70%	0	15
Had/n't	0.00	0.00	0.00	0.00	0%	0	0
Has/n't	0.00	0.00	0.00	0.00	0%	0	0
Have/n't	0.00	0.00	0.00	0.00	0%	0	0
Is/n't	0.04	0.19	-0.15	0.22	529%	0	1
Might/n't	0.00	0.00	0.00	0.00	0%	0	0
Must/n't	0.00	0.00	0.00	0.00	0%	0	0
No	2.86	2.82	0.03	5.68	99%	0	11
Nope	0.21	0.50	-0.28	0.71	233%	0	2
Not	1.46	1.62	-0.16	3.09	111%	0	5
Should/n't	0.00	0.00	0.00	0.00	0%	0	0
Uhuh	0.86	1.53	-0.68	2.39	179%	0	5
Was/n't	0.25	0.65	-0.40	0.90	258%	0	3
Were/n't	0.04	0.19	-0.15	0.22	529%	0	1
Won't	0.36	0.83	-0.47	1.18	231%	0	4
Would/n't	0.32	0.67	-0.35	0.99	208%	0	3

Modals	Mean	SD	SD–	SD+	%SD	R–	R+
Can	2.32	2.68	-0.36	5.00	116%	0	10
Could	0.93	1.68	-0.75	2.60	181%	0	8
May	0.07	0.38	-0.31	0.45	529%	0	2
Might	0.21	0.50	-0.28	0.71	233%	0	2
Must	0.04	0.19	-0.15	0.22	529%	0	1
Shall	0.00	0.00	0.00	0.00	0%	0	0
Should	0.21	0.42	-0.20	0.63	195%	0	1
Will	0.39	0.88	-0.48	1.27	223%	0	4
Would	0.75	0.97	-0.22	1.72	129%	0	3

Pronouns

Reflexive	Mean	SD	SD–	SD+	%SD	R–	R+
Herself	0.00	0.00	0.00	0.00	0%	0	0
Himself	0.04	0.19	-0.15	0.22	529%	0	1
Itself	0.00	0.00	0.00	0.00	0%	0	0
Myself	0.04	0.19	-0.15	0.22	529%	0	1
Ourselves	0.00	0.00	0.00	0.00	0%	0	0
Themselves	0.00	0.00	0.00	0.00	0%	0	0
Yourself	0.00	0.00	0.00	0.00	0%	0	0
Yourselves	0.00	0.00	0.00	0.00	0%	0	0

Demonstrative	Mean	SD	SD–	SD+	%SD	R–	R+
That	9.18	4.69	4.49	13.87	51%	2	21
These	0.46	0.74	-0.28	1.21	160%	0	2
This	4.11	3.74	0.37	7.84	91%	0	14
Those	0.46	0.64	-0.17	1.10	137%	0	2

Quantifying	Mean	SD	SD–	SD+	%SD	R–	R+
Enough	0.04	0.19	-0.15	0.22	529%	0	1
Few	0.07	0.38	-0.31	0.45	529%	0	1
Little	2.46	2.52	-0.05	4.98	102%	0	12
Many	0.04	0.19	-0.15	0.22	529%	0	1
Much	0.14	0.36	-0.21	0.50	249%	0	1
One	5.39	3.93	1.46	9.32	73%	0	14
Several	0.00	0.00	0.00	0.00	0%	0	0

Relative	Mean	SD	SD–	SD+	%SD	R–	R+
What	1.64	1.50	0.15	3.14	91%	0	5
Whatever	0.00	0.00	0.00	0.00	0%	0	0
Which	0.14	0.36	-0.21	0.50	249%	0	1
Whichever	0.00	0.00	0.00	0.00	0%	0	0
Who	0.39	0.63	-0.24	1.02	160%	0	2
Whoever	0.00	0.00	0.00	0.00	0%	0	0
Whom	0.00	0.00	0.00	0.00	0%	0	0
Whose	0.00	0.00	0.00	0.00	0%	0	0

Universal	Mean	SD	SD–	SD+	%SD	R–	R+
All	3.50	2.98	0.52	6.48	85%	0	15
Both	0.14	0.45	-0.31	0.59	314%	0	2
Each	0.07	0.26	-0.19	0.33	367%	0	1
Every	0.21	0.42	-0.20	0.63	195%	0	1
Everybody	0.04	0.19	-0.15	0.22	529%	0	1
Everyone	0.00	0.00	0.00	0.00	0%	0	0
Everything	0.25	0.52	-0.27	0.77	207%	0	2
Everywhere	0.00	0.00	0.00	0.00	0%	0	0

Possessive	Mean	SD	SD–	SD+	%SD	R–	R+
Her	3.04	3.73	-0.69	6.76	123%	0	15
Hers	0.14	0.45	-0.31	0.59	314%	0	2
His	1.79	2.50	-0.71	4.29	140%	0	10
Its	0.00	0.00	0.00	0.00	0%	0	0
Mine	0.29	0.76	-0.48	1.05	267%	0	3
My	3.43	3.43	0.00	6.85	100%	0	10
Our	0.11	0.31	-0.21	0.42	294%	0	1
Ours	0.00	0.00	0.00	0.00	0%	0	0
Their	0.93	1.27	-0.35	2.20	137%	0	5
Theirs	0.00	0.00	0.00	0.00	0%	0	0
Your	0.43	0.69	-0.26	1.12	161%	0	2
Yours	0.04	0.19	-0.15	0.22	529%	0	1

Personal	Mean	SD	SD–	SD+	%SD	R–	R+
He	9.75	8.59	1.16	18.34	88%	0	31
Her	3.04	3.73	-0.69	6.76	123%	0	15
Him	1.75	2.10	-0.35	3.85	120%	0	8
I	16.93	9.23	7.70	26.15	54%	1	36
It	14.43	6.39	8.04	20.82	44%	6	27
Me	0.89	1.29	-0.39	2.18	144%	0	6
She	11.71	9.01	2.71	20.72	77%	0	31
Them	1.86	1.86	0.00	3.72	100%	0	8
They	8.61	5.86	2.75	14.47	68%	1	23
Us	0.07	0.38	-0.31	0.45	529%	0	2
We	1.46	1.48	-0.01	2.94	101%	0	4
You	5.89	5.96	-0.07	11.86	101%	0	26

Partitive	Mean	SD	SD–	SD+	%SD	R–	R+
Any	0.54	1.00	-0.46	1.54	187%	0	3
Anybody	0.00	0.00	0.00	0.00	0%	0	0
Anyone	0.00	0.00	0.00	0.00	0%	0	0
Anything	0.21	0.57	-0.35	0.78	265%	0	2
Anywhere	0.00	0.00	0.00	0.00	0%	0	0
Either	0.07	0.26	-0.19	0.33	367%	0	1
Neither	0.04	0.19	-0.15	0.22	529%	0	1
Nobody	0.11	0.31	-0.21	0.42	294%	0	1
None	0.04	0.19	-0.15	0.22	529%	0	1
No one	0.18	0.48	-0.30	0.65	266%	0	2
Nothing	0.39	0.83	-0.44	1.22	212%	0	3
Some	1.71	1.94	-0.23	3.66	113%	0	7
Somebody	1.29	2.49	-1.21	3.78	194%	0	9
Someone	1.07	2.21	-1.14	3.28	206%	0	9
Someplace	0.04	0.19	-0.15	0.22	529%	0	1
Something	0.39	0.74	-0.34	1.13	188%	0	2

Word List Summary / 6-Year-Olds

(Narration: 100 Utterance Samples N=35)

Questions

	Mean	SD	SD–	SD+	%SD	R–	R+
How	0.11	0.40	-0.29	0.52	353%	0	2
What	2.00	2.83	-0.83	4.83	141%	0	14
When	0.14	0.43	-0.29	0.57	301%	0	2
Where	0.17	0.51	-0.34	0.69	300%	0	2
Which	0.03	0.17	-0.14	0.20	592%	0	1
Who	0.23	0.69	-0.46	0.92	302%	0	3
Whose	0.00	0.00	0.00	0.00	0%	0	0
Why	0.29	0.71	-0.42	1.00	249%	0	3

Conjunctions

	Mean	SD	SD–	SD+	%SD	R–	R+
After	0.31	0.76	-0.44	1.07	241%	0	3
And	34.17	16.22	17.95	50.39	47%	4	74
As	0.31	0.68	-0.36	0.99	215%	0	2
Because	2.57	2.55	0.02	5.12	99%	0	11
But	4.34	3.96	0.39	8.30	91%	0	12
If	0.49	0.82	-0.33	1.30	168%	0	3
Or	0.69	1.16	-0.47	1.84	169%	0	6
Since	0.00	0.00	0.00	0.00	0%	0	0
So	3.57	3.94	-0.36	7.51	110%	0	14
Then	14.09	10.82	3.27	24.91	77%	1	52
Until	0.14	0.43	-0.29	0.57	301%	0	2
While	0.11	0.32	-0.21	0.44	282%	0	1

Negatives

	Mean	SD	SD–	SD+	%SD	R–	R+
Ain't	0.09	0.37	-0.29	0.46	436%	0	2
Are/n't	0.00	0.00	0.00	0.00	0%	0	0
Can/'t	1.34	1.86	-0.52	3.20	139%	0	8
Could/n't	0.57	0.85	-0.28	1.42	149%	0	3
Did/n't	1.37	1.77	-0.40	3.14	129%	0	8
Does/n't	0.26	0.56	-0.30	0.82	218%	0	2
Don't	4.83	3.98	0.85	8.81	82%	0	14
Had/n't	0.00	0.00	0.00	0.00	0%	0	0
Has/n't	0.00	0.00	0.00	0.00	0%	0	0
Have/n't	0.09	0.51	-0.42	0.59	592%	0	3
Is/n't	0.03	0.17	-0.14	0.20	592%	0	1
Might/n't	0.00	0.00	0.00	0.00	0%	0	0
Must/n't	0.00	0.00	0.00	0.00	0%	0	0
No	2.97	2.58	0.39	5.56	87%	0	12
Nope	0.26	0.51	-0.25	0.76	197%	0	2
Not	1.37	1.21	0.16	2.59	89%	0	4
Should/n't	0.00	0.00	0.00	0.00	0%	0	0
Uhuh	1.23	1.54	-0.31	2.76	125%	0	5
Was/n't	0.40	1.22	-0.82	1.62	304%	0	6
Were/n't	0.09	0.37	-0.29	0.46	436%	0	2
Won't	0.20	0.47	-0.27	0.67	236%	0	2
Would/n't	0.17	0.45	-0.28	0.62	264%	0	2

Modals

	Mean	SD	SD–	SD+	%SD	R–	R+
Can	2.60	2.64	-0.04	5.24	101%	0	10
Could	1.17	1.42	-0.25	2.60	122%	0	6
May	0.06	0.34	-0.28	0.40	592%	0	2
Might	0.17	0.38	-0.21	0.55	223%	0	1
Must	0.00	0.00	0.00	0.00	0%	0	0
Shall	0.00	0.00	0.00	0.00	0%	0	0
Should	0.11	0.40	-0.29	0.52	353%	0	2
Will	0.26	0.92	-0.66	1.18	357%	0	5
Would	0.66	1.55	-0.89	2.21	236%	0	8

Pronouns

Reflexive

	Mean	SD	SD–	SD+	%SD	R–	R+
Herself	0.00	0.00	0.00	0.00	0%	0	0
Himself	0.03	0.17	-0.14	0.20	592%	0	1
Itself	0.00	0.00	0.00	0.00	0%	0	0
Myself	0.06	0.24	-0.18	0.29	412%	0	1
Ourselves	0.00	0.00	0.00	0.00	0%	0	0
Themselves	0.00	0.00	0.00	0.00	0%	0	0
Yourself	0.00	0.00	0.00	0.00	0%	0	0
Yourselves	0.00	0.00	0.00	0.00	0%	0	0

Demonstrative

	Mean	SD	SD–	SD+	%SD	R–	R+
That	8.66	4.06	4.60	12.72	47%	1	16
These	0.49	0.78	-0.30	1.27	161%	0	3
This	3.80	3.89	-0.09	7.69	102%	0	13
Those	0.14	0.43	-0.29	0.57	301%	0	2

Quantifying

	Mean	SD	SD–	SD+	%SD	R–	R+
Enough	0.03	0.17	-0.14	0.20	592%	0	1
Few	0.06	0.34	-0.28	0.40	592%	0	2
Little	3.09	3.30	-0.22	6.39	107%	0	13
Many	0.06	0.24	-0.18	0.29	412%	0	1
Much	0.20	0.58	-0.38	0.78	292%	0	3
One	4.54	2.91	1.63	7.46	64%	0	13
Several	0.00	0.00	0.00	0.00	0%	0	0

Relative

	Mean	SD	SD–	SD+	%SD	R–	R+
What	1.66	1.71	-0.06	3.37	103%	0	6
Whatever	0.14	0.49	-0.35	0.64	346%	0	2
Which	0.11	0.40	-0.29	0.52	353%	0	2
Whichever	0.00	0.00	0.00	0.00	0%	0	0
Who	0.20	0.58	-0.38	0.78	292%	0	3
Whoever	0.00	0.00	0.00	0.00	0%	0	0
Whom	0.00	0.00	0.00	0.00	0%	0	0
Whose	0.00	0.00	0.00	0.00	0%	0	0

Universal

	Mean	SD	SD–	SD+	%SD	R–	R+
All	4.97	3.49	1.49	8.46	70%	1	14
Both	0.06	0.24	-0.18	0.29	412%	0	1
Each	0.03	0.17	-0.14	0.20	592%	0	1
Every	0.09	0.37	-0.29	0.46	436%	0	2
Everybody	0.11	0.32	-0.21	0.44	282%	0	1
Everyone	0.00	0.00	0.00	0.00	0%	0	0
Everything	0.14	0.55	-0.41	0.69	385%	0	3
Everywhere	0.03	0.17	-0.14	0.20	592%	0	1

Possessive

	Mean	SD	SD–	SD+	%SD	R–	R+
Her	4.17	4.09	0.08	8.26	98%	0	14
Hers	0.09	0.28	-0.20	0.37	331%	0	1
His	2.54	3.04	-0.50	5.59	120%	0	13
Its	0.03	0.17	-0.14	0.20	592%	0	1
Mine	0.17	0.62	-0.45	0.79	360%	0	3
My	4.54	3.97	0.57	8.52	87%	0	14
Our	0.20	0.47	-0.27	0.67	236%	0	2
Ours	0.00	0.00	0.00	0.00	0%	0	0
Their	1.06	1.11	-0.05	2.17	105%	0	4
Theirs	0.00	0.00	0.00	0.00	0%	0	0
Your	0.40	0.98	-0.58	1.38	244%	0	5
Yours	0.00	0.00	0.00	0.00	0%	0	0

Personal

	Mean	SD	SD–	SD+	%SD	R–	R+
He	12.43	9.20	3.23	21.63	74%	0	43
Her	4.17	4.09	0.08	8.26	98%	0	14
Him	2.66	2.65	0.01	5.30	100%	0	9
I	18.74	8.74	10.00	27.49	47%	2	38
It	14.34	6.85	7.49	21.19	48%	4	32
Me	2.00	2.67	-0.67	4.67	133%	0	14
She	12.57	8.03	4.54	20.61	64%	0	35
Them	1.54	1.69	-0.14	3.23	109%	0	8
They	7.31	4.36	2.96	11.67	60%	0	18
Us	0.14	0.55	-0.41	0.69	385%	0	3
We	1.69	1.97	-0.28	3.65	117%	0	6
You	3.94	3.27	0.67	7.21	83%	0	13

Partitive

	Mean	SD	SD–	SD+	%SD	R–	R+
Any	0.54	1.07	-0.52	1.61	196%	0	5
Anybody	0.00	0.00	0.00	0.00	0%	0	0
Anyone	0.00	0.00	0.00	0.00	0%	0	0
Anything	0.14	0.55	-0.41	0.69	385%	0	3
Anywhere	0.00	0.00	0.00	0.00	0%	0	0
Either	0.17	0.45	-0.28	0.62	264%	0	2
Neither	0.00	0.00	0.00	0.00	0%	0	0
Nobody	0.20	0.53	-0.33	0.73	266%	0	2
None	0.09	0.28	-0.20	0.37	331%	0	1
No one	0.20	0.41	-0.21	0.61	203%	0	1
Nothing	0.11	0.32	-0.21	0.44	282%	0	1
Some	1.49	1.38	0.11	2.87	93%	0	6
Somebody	1.31	2.67	-1.35	3.98	203%	0	9
Someone	0.74	1.60	-0.85	2.34	215%	0	8
Someplace	0.00	0.00	0.00	0.00	0%	0	0
Something	0.57	0.78	-0.21	1.35	136%	0	3

(Narration: 100 Utterance Samples N=50)

Questions	Mean	SD	SD–	SD+	%SD	R–	R+
How	0.20	0.53	-0.33	0.73	267%	0	2
What	0.46	0.86	-0.40	1.32	187%	0	4
When	0.08	0.27	-0.19	0.35	343%	0	1
Where	0.16	0.47	-0.31	0.63	292%	0	2
Which	0.00	0.00	0.00	0.00	0%	0	0
Who	0.80	1.80	-1.00	2.60	224%	0	7
Whose	0.00	0.00	0.00	0.00	0%	0	0
Why	0.18	0.48	-0.30	0.66	268%	0	2

Conjunctions	Mean	SD	SD–	SD+	%SD	R–	R+
After	0.56	0.91	-0.35	1.47	162%	0	4
And	54.38	19.35	35.03	73.73	36%	17	92
As	0.36	0.80	-0.44	1.16	223%	0	4
Because	2.50	1.89	0.61	4.39	75%	0	7
But	4.06	2.87	1.19	6.93	71%	0	14
If	0.98	1.52	-0.54	2.50	155%	0	6
Or	0.70	1.09	-0.39	1.79	156%	0	4
Since	0.06	0.24	-0.18	0.30	400%	0	1
So	5.00	5.15	-0.15	10.15	103%	0	18
Then	22.20	12.96	9.24	35.16	58%	2	60
Until	0.18	0.56	-0.38	0.74	311%	0	3
While	0.20	0.40	-0.20	0.60	202%	0	1

Negatives	Mean	SD	SD–	SD+	%SD	R–	R+
Ain't	0.00	0.00	0.00	0.00	0%	0	0
Are/n't	0.04	0.20	-0.16	0.24	495%	0	1
Can/n't	1.36	2.12	-0.76	3.48	156%	0	10
Could/n't	0.34	0.66	-0.32	1.00	194%	0	3
Did/n't	1.08	1.48	-0.40	2.56	137%	0	7
Does/n't	0.44	0.88	-0.44	1.32	201%	0	4
Don't	2.42	2.30	0.12	4.72	95%	0	10
Had/n't	0.00	0.00	0.00	0.00	0%	0	0
Has/n't	0.04	0.20	-0.16	0.24	495%	0	1
Have/n't	0.14	0.53	-0.39	0.67	382%	0	3
Is/n't	0.12	0.39	-0.27	0.51	321%	0	2
Might/n't	0.00	0.00	0.00	0.00	0%	0	0
Must/n't	0.00	0.00	0.00	0.00	0%	0	0
No	1.98	1.77	0.21	3.75	89%	0	9
Nope	0.08	0.27	-0.19	0.35	343%	0	1
Not	1.86	2.07	-0.21	3.93	111%	0	10
Should/n't	0.00	0.00	0.00	0.00	0%	0	0
Uhuh	0.86	1.58	-0.72	2.44	183%	0	8
Was/n't	0.26	0.49	-0.23	0.75	187%	0	2
Were/n't	0.06	0.31	-0.25	0.37	523%	0	2
Won't	0.10	0.30	-0.20	0.40	303%	0	1
Would/n't	0.18	0.44	-0.26	0.62	243%	0	2

Modals	Mean	SD	SD–	SD+	%SD	R–	R+
Can	2.50	2.86	-0.36	5.36	114%	0	11
Could	0.76	0.92	-0.16	1.68	121%	0	3
May	0.12	0.59	-0.47	0.71	495%	0	4
Might	0.12	0.48	-0.36	0.60	400%	0	3
Must	0.06	0.31	-0.25	0.37	523%	0	2
Shall	0.00	0.00	0.00	0.00	0%	0	0
Should	0.16	0.51	-0.35	0.67	318%	0	3
Will	0.32	0.84	-0.52	1.16	264%	0	4
Would	0.82	1.44	-0.62	2.26	175%	0	6

Pronouns

Reflexive	Mean	SD	SD–	SD+	%SD	R–	R+
Herself	0.02	0.14	-0.12	0.16	707%	0	1
Himself	0.02	0.14	-0.12	0.16	707%	0	1
Itself	0.02	0.14	-0.12	0.16	707%	0	1
Myself	0.14	0.53	-0.39	0.67	382%	0	3
Ourselves	0.00	0.00	0.00	0.00	0%	0	0
Themselves	0.00	0.00	0.00	0.00	0%	0	0
Yourself	0.00	0.00	0.00	0.00	0%	0	0
Yourselves	0.00	0.00	0.00	0.00	0%	0	0

Demonstrative	Mean	SD	SD–	SD+	%SD	R–	R+
That	7.98	4.55	3.43	12.53	57%	0	19
These	0.90	1.34	-0.44	2.24	149%	0	5
This	5.30	4.09	1.21	9.39	77%	0	17
Those	0.26	0.56	-0.30	0.82	217%	0	2

Quantifying	Mean	SD	SD–	SD+	%SD	R–	R+
Enough	0.06	0.24	-0.18	0.30	400%	0	1
Few	0.04	0.20	-0.16	0.24	495%	0	1
Little	3.18	3.10	0.08	6.28	97%	0	12
Many	0.14	0.53	-0.39	0.67	382%	0	3
Much	0.24	0.59	-0.35	0.83	246%	0	3
One	5.94	5.02	0.92	10.96	85%	0	25
Several	0.00	0.00	0.00	0.00	0%	0	0

Relative	Mean	SD	SD–	SD+	%SD	R–	R+
What	1.14	1.18	-0.04	2.32	103%	0	4
Whatever	0.12	0.39	-0.27	0.51	321%	0	2
Which	0.14	0.40	-0.26	0.54	289%	0	2
Whichever	0.00	0.00	0.00	0.00	0%	0	0
Who	0.58	0.88	-0.30	1.46	152%	0	4
Whoever	0.08	0.27	-0.19	0.35	343%	0	1
Whom	0.00	0.00	0.00	0.00	0%	0	0
Whose	0.02	0.14	-0.12	0.16	707%	0	1

Universal	Mean	SD	SD–	SD+	%SD	R–	R+
All	4.92	3.97	0.95	8.89	81%	0	21
Both	0.16	0.42	-0.26	0.58	264%	0	2
Each	0.06	0.31	-0.25	0.37	523%	0	2
Every	0.20	0.49	-0.29	0.69	247%	0	2
Everybody	0.32	0.68	-0.36	1.00	214%	0	3
Everyone	0.10	0.58	-0.48	0.68	580%	0	4
Everything	0.26	0.63	-0.37	0.89	243%	0	3
Everywhere	0.04	0.20	-0.16	0.24	495%	0	1

Possessive	Mean	SD	SD–	SD+	%SD	R–	R+
Her	4.86	5.15	-0.29	10.01	106%	0	20
Hers	0.02	0.14	-0.12	0.16	707%	0	1
His	2.38	2.42	-0.04	4.80	102%	0	8
Its	0.00	0.00	0.00	0.00	0%	0	0
Mine	0.22	0.65	-0.43	0.87	295%	0	3
My	5.40	4.99	0.41	10.39	92%	0	17
Our	0.28	0.76	-0.48	1.04	270%	0	3
Ours	0.00	0.00	0.00	0.00	0%	0	0
Their	1.34	1.44	-0.10	2.78	107%	0	6
Theirs	0.00	0.00	0.00	0.00	0%	0	0
Your	0.84	1.28	-0.44	2.12	153%	0	6
Yours	0.00	0.00	0.00	0.00	0%	0	0

Personal	Mean	SD	SD–	SD+	%SD	R–	R+
He	16.26	10.94	5.32	27.20	67%	0	44
Her	4.86	5.15	-0.29	10.01	106%	0	20
Him	2.90	2.58	0.32	5.48	89%	0	10
I	13.84	7.04	6.80	20.88	51%	3	33
It	13.72	5.40	8.32	19.12	39%	5	31
Me	0.96	1.40	-0.44	2.36	146%	0	7
She	15.50	12.00	3.50	27.50	77%	0	49
Them	2.68	2.16	0.52	4.84	81%	0	10
They	13.52	9.33	4.19	22.85	69%	2	48
Us	0.08	0.27	-0.19	0.35	343%	0	1
We	1.14	1.88	-0.74	3.02	165%	0	9
You	4.22	5.41	-1.19	9.63	128%	0	24

Partitive	Mean	SD	SD–	SD+	%SD	R–	R+
Any	0.40	0.70	-0.30	1.10	175%	0	3
Anybody	0.10	0.36	-0.26	0.46	364%	0	2
Anyone	0.02	0.14	-0.12	0.16	707%	0	1
Anything	0.20	0.53	-0.33	0.73	267%	0	3
Anywhere	0.00	0.00	0.00	0.00	0%	0	0
Either	0.16	0.47	-0.31	0.63	292%	0	2
Neither	0.02	0.14	-0.12	0.16	707%	0	1
Nobody	0.24	0.62	-0.38	0.86	260%	0	3
None	0.06	0.24	-0.18	0.30	400%	0	1
No one	0.04	0.20	-0.16	0.24	495%	0	1
Nothing	0.10	0.30	-0.20	0.40	303%	0	1
Some	2.12	1.93	0.19	4.05	91%	0	9
Somebody	1.42	2.90	-1.48	4.32	204%	0	10
Someone	1.24	2.85	-1.61	4.09	230%	0	10
Someplace	0.00	0.00	0.00	0.00	0%	0	0
Something	0.66	1.14	-0.48	1.80	172%	0	6

Word List Summary / 9-Year-Olds
(Narration: 100 Utterance Samples N=27)

Questions	Mean	SD	SD–	SD+	%SD	R–	R+
How	0.11	0.32	-0.21	0.43	288%	0	1
What	0.56	0.58	-0.02	1.13	104%	0	2
When	0.07	0.27	-0.19	0.34	360%	0	1
Where	0.37	0.79	-0.42	1.16	214%	0	3
Which	0.00	0.00	0.00	0.00	0%	0	0
Who	0.70	1.61	-0.91	2.32	229%	0	6
Whose	0.00	0.00	0.00	0.00	0%	0	0
Why	0.19	0.40	-0.21	0.58	214%	0	1

Conjunctions	Mean	SD	SD–	SD+	%SD	R–	R+
After	0.70	1.07	-0.36	1.77	152%	0	4
And	66.70	20.11	46.59	86.82	30%	33	119
As	0.56	0.93	-0.38	1.49	168%	0	3
Because	2.41	2.44	-0.03	4.85	101%	0	7
But	2.74	3.02	-0.28	5.76	110%	0	11
If	1.00	1.44	-0.44	2.44	144%	0	5
Or	1.33	1.36	-0.03	2.69	102%	0	4
Since	0.11	0.32	-0.21	0.43	288%	0	1
So	11.30	6.62	4.68	17.92	59%	1	26
Then	19.93	11.52	8.41	31.44	58%	4	51
Until	0.11	0.32	-0.21	0.43	288%	0	1
While	0.70	1.17	-0.47	1.87	166%	0	4

Negatives	Mean	SD	SD–	SD+	%SD	R–	R+
Ain't	0.04	0.19	-0.16	0.23	520%	0	1
Are/n't	0.00	0.00	0.00	0.00	0%	0	0
Can/'t	0.59	0.97	-0.38	1.56	164%	0	4
Could/n't	0.96	1.74	-0.78	2.71	181%	0	8
Did/n't	1.33	1.52	-0.19	2.85	114%	0	5
Does/n't	0.26	0.66	-0.40	0.92	253%	0	3
Don't	1.56	1.80	-0.25	3.36	116%	0	6
Had/n't	0.00	0.00	0.00	0.00	0%	0	0
Has/n't	0.04	0.19	-0.16	0.23	520%	0	1
Have/n't	0.07	0.27	-0.19	0.34	360%	0	1
Is/n't	0.07	0.38	-0.31	0.46	520%	0	2
Might/n't	0.00	0.00	0.00	0.00	0%	0	0
Must/n't	0.00	0.00	0.00	0.00	0%	0	0
No	1.52	1.48	0.04	3.00	97%	0	6
Nope	0.19	0.48	-0.30	0.67	261%	0	2
Not	1.81	1.66	0.15	3.48	92%	0	5
Should/n't	0.00	0.00	0.00	0.00	0%	0	0
Uhuh	0.22	0.64	-0.42	0.86	288%	0	3
Was/n't	0.30	0.61	-0.31	0.90	205%	0	2
Were/n't	0.11	0.32	-0.21	0.43	288%	0	1
Won't	0.15	0.36	-0.21	0.51	244%	0	1
Would/n't	0.19	0.40	-0.21	0.58	214%	0	1

Modals	Mean	SD	SD–	SD+	%SD	R–	R+
Can	1.59	1.85	-0.25	3.44	116%	0	7
Could	2.07	2.32	-0.25	4.39	112%	0	9
May	0.07	0.38	-0.31	0.46	520%	0	2
Might	0.07	0.27	-0.19	0.34	360%	0	1
Must	0.00	0.00	0.00	0.00	0%	0	0
Shall	0.00	0.00	0.00	0.00	0%	0	0
Should	0.11	0.32	-0.21	0.43	288%	0	1
Will	0.26	0.81	-0.55	1.07	314%	0	4
Would	0.78	1.65	-0.87	2.43	212%	0	7

Pronouns

Reflexive	Mean	SD	SD–	SD+	%SD	R–	R+
Herself	0.26	0.66	-0.40	0.92	253%	0	3
Himself	0.15	0.36	-0.21	0.51	244%	0	1
Itself	0.00	0.00	0.00	0.00	0%	0	0
Myself	0.00	0.00	0.00	0.00	0%	0	0
Ourselves	0.00	0.00	0.00	0.00	0%	0	0
Themselves	0.00	0.00	0.00	0.00	0%	0	0
Yourself	0.00	0.00	0.00	0.00	0%	0	0
Yourselves	0.00	0.00	0.00	0.00	0%	0	0

Demonstrative	Mean	SD	SD–	SD+	%SD	R–	R+
That	8.89	4.96	3.93	13.85	56%	1	23
These	1.15	1.32	-0.17	2.47	115%	0	6
This	6.19	5.74	0.44	11.93	93%	0	17
Those	0.52	0.98	-0.46	1.49	188%	0	3

Quantifying	Mean	SD	SD–	SD+	%SD	R–	R+
Enough	0.07	0.27	-0.19	0.34	360%	0	1
Few	0.07	0.38	-0.31	0.46	520%	0	2
Little	8.04	6.09	1.94	14.13	76%	0	23
Many	0.04	0.19	-0.16	0.23	520%	0	1
Much	0.15	0.46	-0.31	0.60	308%	0	2
One	6.81	5.34	1.48	12.15	78%	0	23
Several	0.00	0.00	0.00	0.00	0%	0	0

Relative	Mean	SD	SD–	SD+	%SD	R–	R+
What	1.81	2.17	-0.35	3.98	119%	0	9
Whatever	0.04	0.19	-0.16	0.23	520%	0	1
Which	0.41	0.89	-0.48	1.30	218%	0	4
Whichever	0.00	0.00	0.00	0.00	0%	0	0
Who	0.74	1.29	-0.55	2.03	174%	0	5
Whoever	0.00	0.00	0.00	0.00	0%	0	0
Whom	0.00	0.00	0.00	0.00	0%	0	0
Whose	0.04	0.19	-0.16	0.23	520%	0	1

Universal	Mean	SD	SD–	SD+	%SD	R–	R+
All	3.59	2.27	1.32	5.87	63%	0	8
Both	0.07	0.27	-0.19	0.34	360%	0	1
Each	0.15	0.36	-0.21	0.51	244%	0	1
Every	0.19	0.62	-0.44	0.81	336%	0	3
Everybody	0.22	0.70	-0.48	0.92	314%	0	3
Everyone	0.04	0.19	-0.16	0.23	520%	0	1
Everything	0.19	0.48	-0.30	0.67	261%	0	2
Everywhere	0.00	0.00	0.00	0.00	0%	0	0

Possessive	Mean	SD	SD–	SD+	%SD	R–	R+
Her	4.41	5.43	-1.02	9.84	123%	0	18
Hers	0.00	0.00	0.00	0.00	0%	0	0
His	4.19	4.45	-0.26	8.63	106%	0	17
Its	0.00	0.00	0.00	0.00	0%	0	0
Mine	0.67	1.69	-1.02	2.35	253%	0	6
My	7.00	4.89	2.11	11.89	70%	0	19
Our	0.70	0.91	-0.21	1.62	130%	0	3
Ours	0.00	0.00	0.00	0.00	0%	0	0
Their	1.59	1.69	-0.10	3.29	106%	0	6
Theirs	0.00	0.00	0.00	0.00	0%	0	0
Your	1.93	1.54	0.38	3.47	80%	0	5
Yours	0.00	0.00	0.00	0.00	0%	0	0

Personal	Mean	SD	SD–	SD+	%SD	R–	R+
He	24.22	15.01	9.21	39.24	62%	0	55
Her	4.41	5.43	-1.02	9.84	123%	0	18
Him	2.74	2.65	0.09	5.40	97%	0	12
I	11.67	6.11	5.55	17.78	52%	1	23
It	12.70	8.29	4.42	20.99	65%	4	47
Me	2.56	2.58	-0.02	5.13	101%	0	10
She	20.37	11.27	9.10	31.64	55%	0	42
Them	1.85	2.01	-0.16	3.87	109%	0	7
They	11.59	6.94	4.66	18.53	60%	2	31
Us	0.19	0.68	-0.50	0.87	368%	0	3
We	0.70	0.95	-0.25	1.66	135%	0	3
You	5.81	5.13	0.69	10.94	88%	0	21

Partitive	Mean	SD	SD–	SD+	%SD	R–	R+
Any	0.30	0.82	-0.53	1.12	278%	0	4
Anybody	0.07	0.27	-0.19	0.34	360%	0	1
Anyone	0.04	0.19	-0.16	0.23	520%	0	1
Anything	0.33	0.88	-0.54	1.21	263%	0	3
Anywhere	0.04	0.19	-0.16	0.23	520%	0	1
Either	0.15	0.36	-0.21	0.51	244%	0	1
Neither	0.04	0.19	-0.16	0.23	520%	0	1
Nobody	0.59	0.69	-0.10	1.29	117%	0	2
None	0.04	0.19	-0.16	0.23	520%	0	1
No one	0.07	0.38	-0.31	0.46	520%	0	2
Nothing	0.07	0.27	-0.19	0.34	360%	0	1
Some	3.04	2.01	1.03	5.05	66%	0	7
Somebody	2.67	3.70	-1.03	6.37	139%	0	10
Someone	1.70	3.05	-1.34	4.75	179%	0	10
Someplace	0.00	0.00	0.00	0.00	0%	0	0
Something	0.85	1.17	-0.32	2.02	137%	0	4

Word List Summary / 11-Year-Olds

(Narration: 100 Utterance Samples N=27)

Questions

	Mean	SD	SD−	SD+	%SD	R−	R+
How	0.11	0.42	-0.31	0.53	381%	0	2
What	0.15	0.36	-0.21	0.51	244%	0	1
When	0.07	0.27	-0.19	0.34	360%	0	1
Where	0.15	0.60	-0.45	0.75	406%	0	3
Which	0.00	0.00	0.00	0.00	0%	0	0
Who	0.00	0.00	0.00	0.00	0%	0	0
Whose	0.00	0.00	0.00	0.00	0%	0	0
Why	0.00	0.00	0.00	0.00	0%	0	0

Conjunctions

	Mean	SD	SD−	SD+	%SD	R−	R+
After	1.52	1.76	-0.24	3.28	116%	0	8
And	70.26	19.09	51.17	89.35	27%	38	107
As	0.81	1.33	-0.52	2.15	163%	0	4
Because	6.67	5.01	1.66	11.67	75%	0	24
But	5.52	4.19	1.33	9.71	76%	1	16
If	1.04	1.29	-0.25	2.32	124%	0	4
Or	4.81	4.83	-0.01	9.64	100%	0	19
Since	0.07	0.27	-0.19	0.34	360%	0	1
So	10.52	7.39	3.13	17.91	70%	0	31
Then	16.30	8.62	7.67	24.92	53%	3	31
Until	0.26	0.45	-0.19	0.71	172%	0	1
While	0.44	0.80	-0.36	1.25	180%	0	3

Negatives

	Mean	SD	SD−	SD+	%SD	R−	R+
Ain't	0.00	0.00	0.00	0.00	0%	0	0
Are/n't	0.11	0.42	-0.31	0.53	381%	0	2
Can't	1.63	1.67	-0.04	3.30	102%	0	7
Could/n't	0.70	1.23	-0.53	1.94	175%	0	5
Did/n't	2.93	3.33	-0.40	6.25	114%	0	16
Does/n't	0.81	1.14	-0.33	1.96	140%	0	5
Don't	2.11	1.67	0.44	3.78	79%	0	5
Had/n't	0.11	0.42	-0.31	0.53	381%	0	2
Has/n't	0.15	0.46	-0.31	0.60	308%	0	2
Have/n't	0.15	0.36	-0.21	0.51	244%	0	1
Is/n't	0.04	0.19	-0.16	0.23	520%	0	1
Might/n't	0.00	0.00	0.00	0.00	0%	0	0
Must/n't	0.00	0.00	0.00	0.00	0%	0	0
No	1.59	1.65	-0.05	3.24	103%	0	6
Nope	0.00	0.00	0.00	0.00	0%	0	0
Not	1.44	1.19	0.26	2.63	82%	0	5
Should/n't	0.00	0.00	0.00	0.00	0%	0	0
Uhuh	0.07	0.27	-0.19	0.34	360%	0	1
Was/n't	0.81	1.30	-0.49	2.12	160%	0	6
Were/n't	0.11	0.32	-0.21	0.43	288%	0	1
Won't	0.15	0.53	-0.39	0.68	360%	0	2
Would/n't	0.33	0.62	-0.29	0.95	186%	0	2

Modals

	Mean	SD	SD−	SD+	%SD	R−	R+
Can	2.85	2.84	0.01	5.69	100%	0	13
Could	1.52	2.05	-0.53	3.56	135%	0	7
May	0.04	0.19	-0.16	0.23	520%	0	1
Might	0.15	0.46	-0.31	0.60	308%	0	2
Must	0.11	0.58	-0.47	0.69	520%	0	3
Shall	0.00	0.00	0.00	0.00	0%	0	0
Should	0.04	0.19	-0.16	0.23	520%	0	1
Will	0.33	0.62	-0.29	0.95	186%	0	2
Would	1.37	1.69	-0.32	3.06	123%	0	6

Pronouns

Reflexive

	Mean	SD	SD−	SD+	%SD	R−	R+
Herself	0.00	0.00	0.00	0.00	0%	0	0
Himself	0.26	0.59	-0.34	0.85	229%	0	2
Itself	0.04	0.19	-0.16	0.23	520%	0	1
Myself	0.04	0.19	-0.16	0.23	520%	0	1
Ourselves	0.00	0.00	0.00	0.00	0%	0	0
Themselves	0.00	0.00	0.00	0.00	0%	0	0
Yourself	0.00	0.00	0.00	0.00	0%	0	0
Yourselves	0.00	0.00	0.00	0.00	0%	0	0

Demonstrative

	Mean	SD	SD−	SD+	%SD	R−	R+
That	14.93	5.72	9.21	20.64	38%	6	27
These	2.44	2.53	-0.09	4.98	104%	0	9
This	9.52	7.19	2.33	16.70	75%	1	27
Those	0.56	0.85	-0.29	1.40	153%	0	3

Quantifying

	Mean	SD	SD−	SD+	%SD	R−	R+
Enough	0.11	0.32	-0.21	0.43	288%	0	1
Few	0.19	0.48	-0.30	0.67	261%	0	2
Little	1.96	2.16	-0.19	4.12	110%	0	7
Many	0.22	0.58	-0.36	0.80	260%	0	2
Much	0.48	0.70	-0.22	1.18	145%	0	2
One	5.93	4.61	1.32	10.53	78%	0	19
Several	0.00	0.00	0.00	0.00	0%	0	0

Relative

	Mean	SD	SD−	SD+	%SD	R−	R+
What	2.56	2.01	0.55	4.56	79%	0	7
Whatever	0.52	0.94	-0.42	1.45	180%	0	3
Which	0.63	1.28	-0.65	1.91	203%	0	4
Whichever	0.00	0.00	0.00	0.00	0%	0	0
Who	1.37	1.57	-0.20	2.94	115%	0	5
Whoever	0.04	0.19	-0.16	0.23	520%	0	1
Whom	0.00	0.00	0.00	0.00	0%	0	0
Whose	0.04	0.19	-0.16	0.23	520%	0	1

Universal

	Mean	SD	SD−	SD+	%SD	R−	R+
All	6.41	4.88	1.53	11.28	76%	1	22
Both	0.11	0.32	-0.21	0.43	288%	0	1
Each	0.33	0.55	-0.22	0.89	166%	0	2
Every	0.30	0.47	-0.17	0.76	157%	0	1
Everybody	0.52	1.01	-0.50	1.53	196%	0	4
Everyone	0.15	0.46	-0.31	0.60	308%	0	2
Everything	1.48	2.69	-1.21	4.18	182%	0	10
Everywhere	0.00	0.00	0.00	0.00	0%	0	0

Possessive

	Mean	SD	SD−	SD+	%SD	R−	R+
Her	7.15	10.25	-3.10	17.39	143%	0	51
Hers	0.00	0.00	0.00	0.00	0%	0	0
His	7.37	4.83	2.54	12.20	66%	0	17
Its	0.00	0.00	0.00	0.00	0%	0	0
Mine	0.11	0.58	-0.47	0.69	520%	0	3
My	1.59	2.74	-1.14	4.33	172%	0	13
Our	0.26	0.45	-0.19	0.71	172%	0	1
Ours	0.00	0.00	0.00	0.00	0%	0	0
Their	1.96	2.58	-0.62	4.54	131%	0	11
Theirs	0.00	0.00	0.00	0.00	0%	0	0
Your	0.15	0.36	-0.21	0.51	244%	0	1
Yours	0.00	0.00	0.00	0.00	0%	0	0

Personal

	Mean	SD	SD−	SD+	%SD	R−	R+
He	32.04	16.07	15.96	48.11	50%	0	76
Her	7.15	10.25	-3.10	17.39	143%	0	51
Him	7.33	4.51	2.82	11.85	62%	0	15
I	12.48	7.09	5.39	19.57	57%	3	29
It	19.07	7.78	11.30	26.85	41%	8	38
Me	0.56	0.75	-0.20	1.31	135%	0	2
She	13.11	17.68	-4.57	30.79	135%	0	83
Them	4.44	3.41	1.03	7.86	77%	0	16
They	22.26	9.69	12.57	31.95	44%	5	39
Us	0.00	0.00	0.00	0.00	0%	0	0
We	1.04	1.09	-0.05	2.13	105%	0	4
You	4.07	3.76	0.31	7.84	92%	0	15

Partitive

	Mean	SD	SD−	SD+	%SD	R−	R+
Any	0.67	1.00	-0.33	1.67	150%	0	4
Anybody	0.00	0.00	0.00	0.00	0%	0	0
Anyone	0.00	0.00	0.00	0.00	0%	0	0
Anything	0.78	1.31	-0.53	2.09	169%	0	5
Anywhere	0.00	0.00	0.00	0.00	0%	0	0
Either	0.19	0.40	-0.21	0.58	214%	0	1
Neither	0.00	0.00	0.00	0.00	0%	0	0
Nobody	0.04	0.19	-0.16	0.23	520%	0	1
None	0.04	0.19	-0.16	0.23	520%	0	1
No one	0.00	0.00	0.00	0.00	0%	0	0
Nothing	0.11	0.42	-0.31	0.53	381%	0	2
Some	1.56	1.25	0.30	2.81	80%	0	4
Somebody	0.30	0.72	-0.43	1.02	244%	0	3
Someone	0.48	0.80	-0.32	1.28	167%	0	3
Someplace	0.15	0.36	-0.21	0.51	244%	0	1
Something	2.93	3.34	-0.41	6.26	114%	0	15

Word List Summary / 13-Year-Olds
(Narration: 100 Utterance Samples N=27)

Questions	Mean	SD	SD–	SD+	%SD	R–	R+
How	0.00	0.00	0.00	0.00	0%	0	0
What	0.44	0.58	-0.13	1.02	130%	0	2
When	0.00	0.00	0.00	0.00	0%	0	0
Where	0.07	0.27	-0.19	0.34	360%	0	1
Which	0.04	0.19	-0.16	0.23	520%	0	1
Who	0.11	0.42	-0.31	0.53	381%	0	2
Whose	0.00	0.00	0.00	0.00	0%	0	0
Why	0.00	0.00	0.00	0.00	0%	0	0

Conjunctions	Mean	SD	SD–	SD+	%SD	R–	R+
After	1.37	1.39	-0.02	2.76	101%	0	4
And	65.78	15.69	50.09	81.47	24%	36	95
As	0.85	1.03	-0.17	1.88	121%	0	4
Because	5.37	2.94	2.43	8.31	55%	1	11
But	5.52	4.23	1.29	9.75	77%	1	16
If	0.52	0.70	-0.18	1.22	135%	0	2
Or	4.30	5.43	-1.13	9.72	126%	0	28
Since	0.07	0.27	-0.19	0.34	360%	0	1
So	11.07	7.95	3.12	19.03	72%	0	31
Then	13.22	7.36	5.87	20.58	56%	1	25
Until	0.07	0.27	-0.19	0.34	360%	0	1
While	0.33	0.83	-0.50	1.17	250%	0	4

Negatives	Mean	SD	SD–	SD+	%SD	R–	R+
Ain't	0.00	0.00	0.00	0.00	0%	0	0
Are/n't	0.04	0.19	-0.16	0.23	520%	0	1
Can/'t	1.22	1.34	-0.12	2.56	110%	0	5
Could/n't	0.74	0.76	-0.02	1.50	103%	0	2
Did/n't	2.33	2.00	0.33	4.33	86%	0	8
Does/n't	0.56	0.80	-0.25	1.36	144%	0	3
Don't	3.22	2.34	0.88	5.56	73%	1	11
Had/n't	0.04	0.19	-0.16	0.23	520%	0	1
Has/n't	0.04	0.19	-0.16	0.23	520%	0	1
Have/n't	0.30	0.47	-0.17	0.76	157%	0	1
Is/n't	0.07	0.27	-0.19	0.34	360%	0	1
Might/n't	0.00	0.00	0.00	0.00	0%	0	0
Must/n't	0.00	0.00	0.00	0.00	0%	0	0
No	1.52	1.74	-0.22	3.26	115%	0	6
Nope	0.00	0.00	0.00	0.00	0%	0	0
Not	1.37	1.31	0.07	2.68	95%	0	4
Should/n't	0.04	0.19	-0.16	0.23	520%	0	1
Uhuh	0.41	0.80	-0.39	1.20	196%	0	3
Was/n't	0.44	0.75	-0.31	1.20	169%	0	2
Were/n't	0.11	0.32	-0.21	0.43	288%	0	1
Won't	0.07	0.27	-0.19	0.34	360%	0	1
Would/n't	0.44	0.75	-0.31	1.20	169%	0	3

Modals	Mean	SD	SD–	SD+	%SD	R–	R+
Can	1.85	1.85	0.00	3.71	100%	0	7
Could	1.78	1.58	0.20	3.35	89%	0	6
May	0.07	0.38	-0.31	0.46	520%	0	2
Might	0.04	0.19	-0.16	0.23	520%	0	1
Must	0.04	0.19	-0.16	0.23	520%	0	1
Shall	0.00	0.00	0.00	0.00	0%	0	0
Should	0.04	0.19	-0.16	0.23	520%	0	1
Will	0.11	0.32	-0.21	0.43	288%	0	1
Would	1.81	2.48	-0.67	4.30	137%	0	10

Pronouns

Reflexive	Mean	SD	SD–	SD+	%SD	R–	R+
Herself	0.11	0.32	-0.21	0.43	288%	0	1
Himself	0.15	0.46	-0.31	0.60	308%	0	2
Itself	0.00	0.00	0.00	0.00	0%	0	0
Myself	0.00	0.00	0.00	0.00	0%	0	0
Ourselves	0.00	0.00	0.00	0.00	0%	0	0
Themselves	0.07	0.27	-0.19	0.34	360%	0	1
Yourself	0.00	0.00	0.00	0.00	0%	0	0
Yourselves	0.00	0.00	0.00	0.00	0%	0	0

Demonstrative	Mean	SD	SD–	SD+	%SD	R–	R+
That	14.33	7.99	6.35	22.32	56%	5	34
These	2.93	3.06	-0.14	5.99	105%	0	11
This	11.26	6.66	4.60	17.92	59%	0	30
Those	0.11	0.32	-0.21	0.43	288%	0	1

Quantifying	Mean	SD	SD–	SD+	%SD	R–	R+
Enough	0.07	0.27	-0.19	0.34	360%	0	1
Few	0.07	0.38	-0.31	0.46	520%	0	2
Little	1.48	2.19	-0.71	3.67	148%	0	8
Many	0.11	0.32	-0.21	0.43	288%	0	1
Much	0.67	0.88	-0.21	1.54	132%	0	3
One	7.37	3.39	3.98	10.76	46%	3	14
Several	0.00	0.00	0.00	0.00	0%	0	0

Relative	Mean	SD	SD–	SD+	%SD	R–	R+
What	2.00	2.47	-0.47	4.47	123%	0	9
Whatever	0.70	1.38	-0.68	2.09	196%	0	5
Which	0.19	0.40	-0.21	0.58	214%	0	1
Whichever	0.04	0.19	-0.16	0.23	520%	0	1
Who	1.41	1.67	-0.26	3.08	119%	0	6
Whoever	0.00	0.00	0.00	0.00	0%	0	0
Whom	0.00	0.00	0.00	0.00	0%	0	0
Whose	0.00	0.00	0.00	0.00	0%	0	0

Universal	Mean	SD	SD–	SD+	%SD	R–	R+
All	6.44	4.67	1.78	11.11	72%	1	19
Both	0.56	1.01	-0.46	1.57	182%	0	4
Each	0.41	0.93	-0.52	1.34	228%	0	4
Every	0.15	0.46	-0.31	0.60	308%	0	2
Everybody	0.52	0.64	-0.12	1.16	124%	0	2
Everyone	0.07	0.27	-0.19	0.34	360%	0	1
Everything	2.22	3.17	-0.94	5.39	142%	0	12
Everywhere	0.00	0.00	0.00	0.00	0%	0	0

Possessive	Mean	SD	SD–	SD+	%SD	R–	R+
Her	8.56	8.66	-0.10	17.21	101%	0	33
Hers	0.04	0.19	-0.16	0.23	520%	0	1
His	5.30	4.12	1.17	9.42	78%	0	17
Its	0.04	0.19	-0.16	0.23	520%	0	1
Mine	0.15	0.53	-0.39	0.68	360%	0	2
My	0.85	1.32	-0.47	2.17	155%	0	4
Our	0.00	0.00	0.00	0.00	0%	0	0
Ours	0.00	0.00	0.00	0.00	0%	0	0
Their	1.63	2.29	-0.66	3.92	140%	0	8
Theirs	0.04	0.19	-0.16	0.23	520%	0	1
Your	0.19	0.62	-0.44	0.81	336%	0	3
Yours	0.00	0.00	0.00	0.00	0%	0	0

Personal	Mean	SD	SD–	SD+	%SD	R–	R+
He	26.15	14.98	11.17	41.13	57%	10	64
Her	8.56	8.66	-0.10	17.21	101%	0	33
Him	5.89	5.56	0.33	11.45	94%	0	23
I	12.63	7.14	5.49	19.77	57%	2	32
It	20.11	10.78	9.33	30.89	54%	4	56
Me	0.70	0.95	-0.25	1.66	135%	0	3
She	14.48	11.99	2.49	26.47	83%	0	39
Them	4.93	3.12	1.80	8.05	63%	1	12
They	22.48	12.95	9.53	35.44	58%	1	55
Us	0.04	0.19	-0.16	0.23	520%	0	1
We	0.93	1.00	-0.07	1.92	108%	0	4
You	6.59	8.11	-1.52	14.70	123%	0	33

Partitive	Mean	SD	SD–	SD+	%SD	R–	R+
Any	0.56	1.12	-0.57	1.68	202%	0	5
Anybody	0.22	0.51	-0.28	0.73	228%	0	2
Anyone	0.04	0.19	-0.16	0.23	520%	0	1
Anything	0.78	1.01	-0.23	1.79	130%	0	3
Anywhere	0.00	0.00	0.00	0.00	0%	0	0
Either	0.07	0.38	-0.31	0.46	520%	0	2
Neither	0.07	0.27	-0.19	0.34	360%	0	1
Nobody	0.26	0.45	-0.19	0.71	172%	0	1
None	0.00	0.00	0.00	0.00	0%	0	0
No one	0.07	0.38	-0.31	0.46	520%	0	2
Nothing	0.37	0.74	-0.37	1.11	200%	0	2
Some	1.37	1.28	0.09	2.65	93%	0	5
Somebody	0.04	0.19	-0.16	0.23	520%	0	1
Someone	0.07	0.27	-0.19	0.34	360%	0	1
Someplace	0.00	0.00	0.00	0.00	0%	0	0
Something	2.52	3.36	-0.84	5.87	133%	0	17

Software Information

*Language Analysis Software**

	Strategic Analysis of Language Transcripts (SALT I and II)	Computerized Profiling (CP) Mac and IBM Versions	Pye Analysis of Language (PAL)
Analyses Available	Brown's Stage Analysis MLU TTR Number of Total Words Number of Different Words Pauses (within and between utterances) Maze Analysis Word and Utterance per Minute Transcript summary information Distribution by speaker turns Utterance and maze distribution tables Word and morpheme tables Code tables Code and lexical search: 1. by word or code list 2. exact match—"logical strings" 3. "next to" or "in order" strings	Bloom and Lahey (modified) Conversational Act Profile (CAP) Developmental Sentence Scoring (DSS) Language Assessment, Remediation, and Sampling Procedure (LARSP) Mean Length of Utterance (MLU) Profile in Semantics-Lexical (PRISM-L) Profile of Prosody (PROP) Type Token Ratio (TTR) Profile of Phonology (PROPH) on IBM version Concordance of phrase-level categories Constituent or lexical search Early Vocabularies Picture Elicited Screening Procedure (PESP) on IBM version Verb Valency Verb-form profile LARSP Learning module Reliability analysis for LARSP, DSS, PRISM-L Reads and writes SALT- and CAP-formatted transcript files (automated conversion from SALT to CP)	MLU Procedures for Phonological Analysis of Children's Language, Ingram (1981) Analysis of Prepositions (APRON) Sentence type classification Sentential productivity Lexical concordance Syntactic concordance Automated conversion from SALT to PAL
User-Defined Features	Coding scheme is user defined Word and code lists used in automatic searches may be changed Additional characters may be legalized in transcript files Certain default displays may be changed	All dictionaries utilized by program may be changed LARSP error categories may be changed	Coding scheme is user defined
Hardware Needed	Monitor, printer, disk file (+)IBM-compatible with 640K RAM Floppy or hard drive Apple II Mac version soon to be completed	Monitor, printer, disk file Macintosh Plus or better hard drive or (+)IBM-compatible with 256K RAM 2 floppy drives or hard drive	Monitor#, printer#, disk file# IBM-compatible with 256K RAM floppy or hard drive
Purchasing Information	Language Analysis Laboratory Waisman Center on Mental Retardation and Human Development University of Wisconsin-Madison Madison, WI 53706 USA	US $100 Computerized Profiling c/o Department of Speech Pathology and Audiology Ithaca College Ithaca, NY 14850 USA	US $45 Clifton Pye 200 Arrowhead Drive Lawrence, KS 66049 USA

---

* Table adapted from Dr. Steven H. Long, Ph.D., Department of Speech Pathology, Ithaca College, Ithaca, NY
(+) Recommended
All output is as text files, which may be viewed or printed from DOS or word processor program

What Information Will SALT Provide?

SALT offers options for a variety of pre-set analyses as well as user-specified analyses. Some of the information from the pre-set analyses include
- types of utterances including distribution of incomplete, unintelligible, and nonverbal utterances;
- calculation of total number of words, type token ratio (TTR), mean length of utterance (MLU) and Brown's linguistic stage and expected age range;
- number and length of pauses and rate of speaking;
- number, length and distribution of mazes (false starts, repetitions and reformulations) by utterance length;
- alphabetized lists and frequencies of word roots, bound morphemes, and codes;
- distribution of utterances by length in terms of words and morphemes;
- distribution of speaker turns by length in terms of number of utterances;
- standard word lists useful in directing syntactic and semantic analysis by providing frequencies for sets of words, including question words, negatives, conjunctions, modal and semi-auxiliaries, pronouns, and any set of words you define.

In addition to the pre-set analyses, user-specified analyses (called "searches") allow one to select specific words or entries of interest within the transcript. Search speaker, ending punctuation, length of utterance, position within the transcript, and any combination of words, morphemes, or codes present within the utterance. Selected utterances may be viewed, counted coded, printed, stored in a file, or searched again.

SALT Transcript-Entry Conventions*

When entering the transcript, follow the conventions listed below in Sections A through S. Some of the conventions are optional and their use depends entirely on your needs while others are mandatory in order to obtain reliable results.

Type in upper- and/or lower-case letters. Do not number the utterances in your transcript.

As a general rule, if you cannot understand a speaker's utterance after listening to it three times, consider it to be partly unintelligible or completely unintelligible.

Note: When a speaker's utterance is too long to be typed on one line, you must go on to the next line, indent two spaces to line up this continuation with the beginning of the previous utterance, and continue typing. SED, the Salt Editor, does this automatically. You just type the utterances, pressing <ENTER> only once at the end of each utterance. Long utterances will be split and the continuation lines indented automatically.

The last section, Section T, contains a listing of the transcript-entry errors.

* Miller, Jon and Robin Chapman. *Salt: A Computer Program for the Systematic Analysis of Language Transcripts*. Madison, WI: Language Analysis Laboratory, Waisman Center, University of Wisconsin-Madison. © 1991. Reprinted with permission.

A. Labels To Identify The Speakers "$"

1. Two-Speaker Transcripts

In order to differentiate between the utterances of the first and second speaker, a $ label line, which contains an identifying label for each speaker in the transcript, beginning with a dollar ($) symbol, must be entered before the first utterance is entered. It is recommended that it be the first line in the transcript. Place a comma between the two names. You may leave a space between the comma and the second speaker's name. The utterances of the first and second speaker are differentiated by a unique letter entered at the beginning of each utterance which corresponds to the first letter of each entry on the $ label line. The initial letter of each label must be unique since this letter is used to differentiate between the speakers. These names will be used to label the analyses. If either name exceeds five characters, only the first five will be used for labelling. Only the first character of each name must be an alphabet character. If a $ label line is not entered correctly in the transcript, the SALT1 program will terminate and the line must be entered correctly before processing can proceed.

Example of a two-speaker transcript (SALT1 will label the data as BILLY and JANE):

> $ Billy, Jane
> J Kittycat.
> B I see you.
> B You big kitty.

Note: The first speaker does not refer to the first person to speak in the transcript but is arbitrarily assigned to one of the speakers, usually the one of primary focus. The first name entered on the $ label line is referred to as "1st Speaker" and the second name is the "2nd Speaker." In the above example, Billy is the first speaker and Jane is the second speaker.

2. Single Speaker Transcripts

If you are entering the utterances of a single speaker, enter a $ followed by the single speaker's name, before the first utterance of your transcript. If you must enter child utterances, for example, SALT1 will provide all data for the first speaker and print out "zeros" for the absent speaker.

Example of a single speaker line:

> $ Billy

3. Transcripts With More Than Two Speakers

When entering the utterances of more than two speakers, you need to decide how you would like to have the SALT program group them for analysis. SALT can only recognize up to three speaker units but each unit may consist of one or more speakers occurring within the transcript. There are no limits to the number of individual speakers occurring within a single unit. The $ label line may contain from one to three speaker units. All speakers in a transcript must be represented in one (and only one) of the speaker units. Utterances comprising the first speaker unit are summarized as the "1st speaker"; utterances comprising the second speaker unit are summarized as the "2nd speaker"; and utterances comprising the third speaker unit are not included in the analyses. Within a speaker unit, each speaker identifier must be separated by a space; speaker units are separated with a comma. The first letter of each speaker identifier must be unique as it is used to differentiate that speaker from all others. Following are examples of various ways of specifying the multiple speaker units. The participants in this conversation are defined as follows:

> A = first child
> B = second child
> C = mother
> D = father
> E = examiner

Examples of possible combinations:

> $ Achild Bchild, Cmother Dfather, Eexaminer

In this analysis, the first speaker will be A and B combined; second speaker will be C and D combined; and the third speaker will be the E. The utterances of E will be ignored with the exception of the turntaking counts.

> $ Achild, Bchild

In the analyses, the first speaker will be A and the second speaker will be B. Note: This example assumes that speakers C, D and E are not included in this particular transcript.

> $ A B, E, C D

In this analyses, the first speaker will be A and B combined; the second speaker will be E; and the third speaker will be C and D. The third speaker will be ignored for the purposes of the analysis with the exception of speaker turn counts.

B. Timing Information "-"

If you enter the length of the transcript in minutes:seconds, the program will calculate rate based on Total Utterance Attempts/Minute and Total Words in Utterance Attempts/Minute. Enter time in hours:minutes:seconds 00:00:00 or minutes:seconds 00:00 on a line beginning with a hyphen (-). Timing information may be placed periodically throughout the transcript. The timing and rate information in SALT1's transcript summary is based on the last time entered in the transcript. Example of timing entry on a seven minute transcript:

> $ Child, Examr
> - 0:00 {required entry}
> C What are we gonna do?
> E You can play with any toy you want.
> - 7:00

If the timing line entered before the first utterance entry is not in the form 00:00 or 00:00:00, the SALT program automatically subtracts this beginning time from the last time entry. For example, suppose you decide to begin transcribing two minutes into a tape. Enter the following:

```
$  Child Examr
-  2:00
C  What are we gonna do?
E  You can play with any toy you want.
-  3:00
C  I want the truck.
C  I want the red truck.
E  Push the truck.
-  4:00
C  Truck is go/ing fast.
C  Under the bridge.
E  Make the truck go over the bridge.
-  5:00
C  Uhoh, the truck turn/ed over.
```

The transcript began two minutes into the conversation and the last timing entry was at five minutes. All timing and rate information will be based on a transcript time of five minutes less two minutes for a total of three minutes.

You may also want to code clock time within a transcript. Clock time must be in military time with hours from one to 24. The initial start time must be set before the first utterance. Consider, for example, the following example based on clock time. Suppose the transcript began at 11:47:53 and at 11:58:39 the conversation is interrupted while the child gets a drink. It is resumed at 12:03:47 and continues until 12:13:29. The following transcript illustrates the format for this timing:

```
$  Child Examr
-  11:47:52.
M  What are you gonna do?
M  You can play with any toy you want.
C  I want the truck.
C  I want the red truck.
E  Push the truck.
C  I want a drink.
-  11:58:47.
=  Mom and child leave room to get a drink.
-  12:03:39.
M  What do you want to do now?
C  Read a story.
C  Read this story.
-  12:13:29.
```

Rates for this transcript will be based on the beginning time of 11:47:52 minus the final time of 12:13:29 for a total of 25:37, less the time out for a drink of 4:42, for a total time of 20:45.

C. Entering Identification Information "+"

You may want to enter identification information at the beginning of your transcript (or anywhere else in the transcript). This information may include speaker's age, subject number, date of transcript, description of code, etc. Enter such information on a line which is initialized with a plus symbol (+) in the first column. You may enter as many information lines as you like at any point in your transcript. When a SALT1 analysis is run on a transcript which contains plus lines, they are listed together as part of the summary information. It is not necessary to leave a space between the + and the beginning of the entry, however, the beginning of any continuation lines must be indented two spaces from the left margin. Pause time does not affect timing information. The following is an example of identification entries:

```
$  Child, Examr
+  ID LD121.
+  DOB is 7/15/77.
+  Environment child's home with mother present.
+  DOE 6/5/85
E  Are you done with your lunch?
C  Yeah [response].
+  [response]
=  child's response to a question.
```

D. Pauses ":" or ";"

1. Frequency and Duration of Pause-Time Between Utterances

If you are interested in the frequency and duration of pauses which occur between utterances (not within), you may code this information during transcript-entry. Enter the length of the pauses in minutes:seconds on lines which begin with either a colon (:) or a semicolon (;). You may enter a few words to describe the nature of the pause-time immediately following the time entry. If the pause occurs between utterances of two *different* speakers, use a : indicating the end of a speaker turn.

If the pause occurs between utterances of the same speaker, however, use a : if a new speaker turn follows the pause or a ; if a new speaker turn does not follow the pause.

This information is important to the interpretation of the turn length analysis, which is part of the SALT1 summary information. In order to maintain consistency, you should decide what constitutes "pause-time" before beginning to enter transcript. The program does not define a minimum or maximum duration for pause-time; the pause boundaries depend on your coding purposes.

When you run the SALT program, a pause-time summary appears as part of the summary information.

Example of pause-time entry when accompanied by a change in speaker turn:

```
$  Child, Examr
E  Let me answer that telephone.
:  01:03 {telephone call}
E  Sorry for that interruption.
E  It's hard to get Aunt Ruth off the phone!
```

Example of pause-time entry when not accompanied by a change in speaker turn:

```
$  Child, Examr
C  We drive in a car.
;  00:08
C  We don't take an airplane.
```

2. More On Turn Length and Topic-Change

Even if you do not enter pause-times in your transcript, you should still be aware of using the : symbol which is used to disambiguate speaker turn lengths. Suppose you entered a speaker's utterance and then there was a long pause during the telephone call, as depicted above. After the pause, the same speaker (E) resumed talking. If you were not coding pause-times, an example of how you might enter the same utterances would be as follows:

```
$ Child, Examr
E Let me answer that telephone.
= telephone call
E Sorry for the interruption.
E It's hard to get Aunt Ruth off the phone!
```

The problem with the above entry is that the program will interpret the three consecutive utterances by E as a *single* speaking turn, three utterances in length. This does not reflect the actual situation, however, because the telephone call interrupted the speaker turn. One solution to this discrepancy would be to use the : symbol by itself to indicate the cessation of a speaker turn (without having to code the length of the pause if you are not interested in such detail). The only characters which can affect speaker turn are : and a change in speaker identifiers such as E and C. The following entry accurately reflects two different speaker turns, one which is one utterance in length and one which consists of two utterances.

Example of using : to end a speaker turn:

```
$ Child, Examr
E Let me answer that telephone.
:
E Sorry for the interruption.
E It's hard to get Aunt Ruth off the phone!
```

3. Frequency and Duration of Pause-Time Within Utterances

If you are interested in the frequency and duration of pauses occurring within utterances you may code this information by entering the length of the pauses in minutes:seconds or :seconds, within either the main body of the utterance or within a maze. Pause-time should be separated from the remainder of the utterance by spaces. For example:

```
$ Child, Examr
E What movie did you go see?
C It was called (um 0:05 or :5) Ghost Busters.
```

If you are interested in the frequency of pauses but not their lengths, you may enter a colon (:) without time. For example:

```
$ Child Examr
E What movie did you go see?
C It was called (um :) Ghost Busters.
```

E.   Transcriber Comment Lines "="

You may want to enter contextual remarks or describe conversational transitions to improve the readability of the transcript. Enter your comments on a line which begins with an equal (=) symbol. You may enter as many comment lines as you want at any point in the transcript. Identify each new comment line with an = symbol. The use of transcriber's comments does not affect the SALT analysis in any way.

Example of transcriber's comment:

```
$  Child, Examr
E  Where is that thing?
=  E gets up to search for C's jacket.
C  Over here.
```

F.   Comments Within Utterances "{}"

You may use braces {} during transcript-entry to mark information such as gestures, vocalizations, contextual descriptions related to an utterance, etc. The SALT analysis ignores the contents of the {} but SEARCH can retrieve any part of a transcript line or an utterance up to the final marker. You may put anything inside {} but they cannot be nested. Do not place a comment after an utterance-final marker. Although you may use {} to make a comment on any line-type, the use of comments on speaker utterances has special meaning. On speaker utterances, you may either embed a comment within the utterance or you may use a comment on a speaker utterance all by itself. A comment which appears by itself on a speaker line is called a "nonverbal utterance." Nonverbal utterances are typically used to mark communicative gestures which contribute to the speaker turn.

You may use {} to embed single or multiple comments on any transcript line. You should embed comments which relate only to the immediate utterance. Otherwise, you should place the comment on an = line as a transcriber comment. The following is an example of an utterance with a comment:

```
$  Child, Examr
E  Show me the book.
C  There {but points to TV set}.
```

G.   Punctuation Conventions

1. End-of-Utterance Punctuation: Speaker Utterances (A-Z)

Every speaker utterance must end with either . ! ? > or ^. > denotes an abandoned utterance, that is, if the speaker stops in mid-utterance and does not complete the utterance; ^ denotes an interrupted utterance. An example is if the door slams and the speaker's utterance is not completed as a result of the distraction.

2. End-of-Entry Punctuation: Special Character Lines

Special character lines are the non-utterance entries. They begin with one of the following characters ($ + - : ; =) and do not require utterance-final punctuation. You may use final markers (> ? ! . ^) if you want to do so. If a special character line is continued on the following line, the new line must be indented two spaces.

3. Within-Utterance Punctuation

a) Within Words * / [] ' .

The only punctuation marks that can be used within a word are asterisks for omissions, slashes for bound morphemes, braces for morpheme codes, apostrophes, and periods.

b) Between Words , " () {} [] <>

The only punctuation marks that can be used between words are commas, quotations, parentheses () to mark mazes, braces {} for comments, square brackets [] for utterance and morpheme codes, and arrows <> to mark overlap in talking between speakers. Do not use any other punctuation marks or symbols such as $, /, #, etc., unless they are serving as "codes" within square brackets [] or are contained within braces {}.

4. Special Character Lines ($ + - : ; =)

You may use any symbols on special character lines as long as the conventions for special lines are not violated.

H. Codes "[]"

1. General Description

SALT's coding option is one of the most flexible elements of the program. Four different types of codes are available: Utterance Codes, Special Line Codes, Word Codes, and Morpheme Codes. A code consists of certain characters enclosed within square brackets, e.g., [code]. The use of codes does not alter the analysis of the transcript in any fashion.

Codes may be inserted either directly, with the word processor or editor used for transcript-entry, or via the CODE option in SALT2. You may want to code words or utterances that contain errors or irregularities at the time of transcript entry. Just attach a code to the word or utterance in question and go on with your transcription. If you are interested in a more elaborate coding scheme such as coding parts of speech or utterances with specific characteristics, you should insert the codes on a copy of your transcript file after transcript-entry has been completed. The coding power comes from the ability to directly call up those words or utterances through SEARCH in SALT2 and to obtain frequency summaries in SALT1.

While there are special constraints on each type of code, as discussed below, there are conventions which apply to all four types. It is suggested that you define each code used on a + line in the transcript for future reference. It is strongly recommended that your coding system be well defined before you begin inserting codes into your transcript in order to avoid problems with inconsistency in coding which might arise.

2. Utterance Codes

These codes are used only on lines beginning with a speaker identifier. You may insert any number of codes per line, anywhere within the utterance, as long as they precede the end-of-utterance punctuation mark. A code must be completely contained either within the main body of the utterance or within a single maze. Leave a space on both sides of the code unless it is bounded on the right side by an end-of-utterance punctuation mark or on either side by another utterance code.

3. Special-Line Codes

These codes are used only on lines beginning with a special line identifier (+ = ; - or :). You may insert any number of codes per line, anywhere on the line.

4. Word and Morpheme Codes

Word codes are used to mark entire words, and morpheme codes are used to mark word roots or bound morphemes. The only difference between word codes and morpheme codes is their position within the word. They are indistinguishable in the Word/Morpheme Code Tables. The conventions are as follows:

> [code1]root[code2]/inflection[code3][code4]
> where:
> [code1] is a morpheme code that refers to the word root
> [code2] is a morpheme code that refers to the bound morpheme
> [code3] and [code4] are word codes that refer to the entire word (word root plus bound morpheme)

You may insert any number of codes per word, either preceding the root, preceding the bound morpheme, or following the word. Do *not* leave a space between the code and the word, or part of the word, it is marking.

5. Coding Example

Suppose you wanted to code the following features in one or more transcripts to facilitate your analysis:

1. child's use of early- versus late-acquired verbs
2. child's substitution of object pronouns for subject pronouns

Here is one potential way to code this information using utterance codes:

> $ Child, Examr
> E What are you do/ing?
> C Me go[EV] up [OP-SP].
> + [EV] = Early acquired verb
> + [OP-SP] = Object pronoun used for subject.

6. Code Restrictions

a) Do not use more than 24 characters per code.
b) Avoid using symbols which have special meaning in SALT (SALT transcript-entry symbols and SEARCH symbols). Especially avoid using *and* or = as their usage will cause a warning message in SALT1.
c) Do not use a blank space within a code and never split the code between lines.
d) Do not nest codes [[]].

I. Mazes "()"

False starts, repetitions, and reformulations are all grouped together as "mazes." Mazes are coded within parentheses (like this). Words found in mazes are excluded from many of the calculations including "Number of Different Word Roots," "Total Number of Words," and "Mean Length of Utterance (MLU)." It is essential, however, that they conform to the entry conventions required for SALT transcripts as the contents are checked during the error checking routine and are used to produce distribution tables based on the mazes, lists of words or codes found within mazes, and an analysis of the pauses found within mazes. The following is an example:

```
$  Child, Examr.
C  (I like) I like the (um) red one.
C  Not the (bl*, bl*) blue one.
```

J. Overlapping Speech "<>"

Overlapping speech between speakers may be marked by enclosing the overlapping segments in arrows <>. The use of arrows does not affect the analysis in any way. For example:

```
$  Child, Examr.
E  Look at the <circus clown>.
C  <He has> a funny hat.
```

K. Bound Morpheme Conventions "/"

If you want SALT1 to calculate MLU in morphemes, Brown's Stage, Expected Age Range, and provide a Bound Morpheme Table, you must separate each bound morpheme from the free morpheme with a slash (/). Bound morphemes are recognized when they immediately follow a slash without blank spaces. Words cannot begin with slashes. Thus, prefixes cannot be coded as morphemes. You should decide upon what constitutes a bound morpheme for your purposes before entering your transcript. It is suggested that you adopt the following conventions in order to group similar inflections which take on various spellings.

1. Possessive Inflections (-s, -'s)
Use Z so that DAD'S becomes DAD/Z and YOURS becomes YOUR/Z.

2. Plural Noun Inflections (-s, -es)
Use S so that BABIES becomes BABY/S and HOUSES becomes HOUSE/S. Do not mark nouns which only have a plural form, that is, use PANTS, CLOTHES, etc.

3. Plural and Possessive Inflections (-s')
Use S/Z so that BABIES' becomes BABY/S/Z and FATHERS' becomes FATHER/S/Z.

4. Third Person Singular Verb Forms (-s, -es)
Use 3S (for both -s and -es forms) so that GOES becomes GO/3S and TELLS becomes TELL/3S. Note: Use DOES *without* a slash (considered one morpheme).

5. Other Verb Tense Inflections (-ed, -d, -ing)

Use ED (for both -ed and -d forms) so that LOVED becomes LOVE/ED and DIED becomes DIE/ED. Use ING so that DOING becomes DO/ING and HAVING becomes HAVE/ING.

6. Contractible Verb Forms (-'m, -'s, -'ll, -'re, -'ve)

Use the free morpheme root spelling with the contracted verb stem so that I'M becomes I/'M, IT'S becomes IT/'S, YOU'LL becomes YOU/'LL, WE'RE becomes WE/'RE, and THEY'VE becomes THEY/'VE.

7. Negative Contractions (-n't, -'t)

Use the root spelling of the free morpheme followed by /N'T or /'T. DOESN'T becomes DOES/N'T, CAN'T becomes CAN/'T, and DIDN'T becomes DID/N'T. Note: Use DON'T, WON'T, and AIN'T *without* a slash (considered one morpheme).

8. Special Notes

    a) Do not mark irregular verb forms or catenatives as inflections (use DOES, GONNA, etc.).

    b) When the spelling of a free morpheme such as CRY changes with the addition of the bound morpheme, use the root spelling of the free morpheme (as if the bound morpheme is not there). Then, simply add the slash plus the bound morpheme (for example, CRY/ED). If this is not done, the stem CRI will be treated as a different word from CRY and thereby inflate Type Token Ratio (TTR) as well as Number of Different Words.

    c) Words that contain a bound morpheme in an adjectival form which cannot be used in that context without the bound morpheme should be entered without a slash (i.e., scrambled egg, bowling pin, swimming pool).

    d) Do not mark predicate adjectives as inflections (use I AM TIRED; THEY LOOK BORED; THE DOOR IS CLOSED).

    e) Do not mark gerunds as inflections (use SWIMMING IS FUN).

L. Omissions of Words "*word" or Bound Morphemes "/ *bm"

1. Omission of Words in Obligatory Contexts

You may also elect to mark the speaker's omission of any word (for example, auxiliary elements). To do so, place an asterisk (*) at the beginning of the word without skipping a space.

Example of omitted word (child said "He going home"):

      E Where/'s he go/ing?
      C He *is go/ing home.

2. Omission of Bound Morphemes in Obligatory Contexts

You may wish to mark the speaker's failure to use a bound morpheme in an obligatory context. To do so, place an asterisk immediately before the omitted bound morpheme. You still must use the slash.

Example of omitted bound morpheme (child said "Boy go here"):

> E Where does the boy go?
> C Boy go/*3s here.

M. Abandoned ">" or Interrupted "^" Utterances

If a speaker stops in mid-utterance, end that utterance fragment with > and no period. If a speaker is interrupted before completing an utterance, end the utterance fragment with ^ and no period. Any utterance ending either with > or ^ is considered incomplete; any utterance which ends with . ? or ! is considered complete.
Examples of interrupted and abandoned utterances:

> $ Jane, Billy
> J Do you remember>
> J Oh, never mind.
> B Jane, I told you^
> J Come quick!
> B To stop that.

Incomplete and abandoned utterances are included in an analysis based on Total Utterances but not Complete and Intelligible Utterances. Be aware that words in an incomplete or interrupted utterance are not included in the calculation of TTR.

N. Abandoned or Interrupted Words "wor*"

If a speaker is interrupted or abandons an utterance mid-word, either in a maze or at the end of an utterance, enter the portion of the word you can discern followed by an asterisk (*). The incomplete word is considered one word for the word and morpheme counts. For example:

> $ Katie, Steve
> K I want the (bl*, bl*) blue one.
> S I'm using it.
> K But I want th*^
> S No, I need it!

O. Unintelligible Segments "X"

Use X to designate each unintelligible word/syllable. You may type in as many X's in one utterance as are needed. You can use any number of X's. Unintelligible words must consist entirely of X's. Words that just begin or end with X's (for example, "XXer" or "mXXX") are considered intelligible.
Example of unintelligible segments:

> $ C, E
> E Where's the dog going?
> C Go XX now.
> E Did you see the airplane?
> C x x up x.
> C XX.

P. Phonetically Consistent Forms "PCF"

PCF stands for "phonetically consistent form" which is an utterance or part of an utterance that fails to approximate the adult form and does not show consistent application to objects or situations but which tends to be stable in production with a distinct prosody (Fletcher and Garman, 1979).

The PCF convention may be useful for marking the intentional vocalizations normally occurring during the second year of life.

Example of PCF entries (with embedded comments):

> $ Child, Examr
> E Can you see the baby?
> C PCF {sounds like "tata"}.
> C Here PCF {sounds like "baba"}.

Q. Nonverbal Utterances

This convention is used to code a nonverbal conversational turn. Place a description of the nonverbal utterances as a comment within braces {}. The program considers nonverbal utterances to be "zero words in length" for calculation of the Distributional Analyses, part of the Transcript Summary Information. A nonverbal utterance is considered to be an utterance for calculation of speaker turn length, which is also part of the Distributional Analyses.

Example of a nonverbal utterance:

> $ Child, Examr
> E Show me the ball.
> C {points to ball}.
> E Good job!

R. Idiosyncratic Forms "%word"

Type a % mark preceding a word which is used as an idiosyncratic form.
For example:

> See my %vrroom.

In this example, vrroom is used as an idiosyncratic form to represent the word car.

S. Spelling Conventions

Type in the exact words or glosses for each speaker deleting expressions such as "aah," "um," etc. when they are not used as affirmation, negation, or interrogation. Numbers may be entered in written form or expressed as digits. Hyphenated words should appear as one word. Use the following conventions to ensure consistency within each file and between files:

> AIN'T
> ATTA (for "THAT'S A")
> BETCHA (as in "I BETCHA CAN'T DO THAT.")

DOCTOR or DR
GONNA
GOTTA
HAFTA
HEY
HI
HUH (as in requesting clarification)
LET'S
LIKETA
LOOKIT
MHM (as in indicating assent)
MISTER or MR
MISSES or MRS
MISS or MS
NOPE
OOPS
OOPSY
OK (for "OKAY")
OUGHTA (as in "I OUGHTA DO THAT.")
PSST
SPOSTA (for "SUPPOSED TO")
TRYNTA (for "TRYING TO")
UHHUH (as indicating "YES")
UHUH (as indicating "NO")
WANNA
WHATCHA (as in "WHATCHA DOING?")
YEAH (for "YES")
YEP (for a short, clipped "YES")

Note: If 'CUZ is used instead of BECAUSE, enter BECAUSE. If 'YA is used instead of YOU, enter YOU. Do not use an apostrophe at the beginning of a word.

Loban's Analysis of Oral Language*

I. Language Sample

Obtain a continuous narrative of 30 *communication units*. Means of eliciting this include asking child to tell favorite story, TV program episode, etc. See Section Two on sampling. Transcribe the sample.

Loban's decision rules for utterance segmentation were developed to provide a language analysis for children from grades 1 through 12. His goal was to document the relationship between progress in acquiring oral language skills and the acquisition of literacy skills. He segments utterances into what he calls, "communication units." Communication units are defined as an independent clause and its modifiers. A communication unit is an utterance that cannot be further divided without the disappearance of its essential meaning or a subordinate clause that is part of the independent predication. In all cases, the words comprising communication units are either independent grammatical predications or propositions, or answers to questions which lack only the repetition of the question elements to satisfy the criterion of independent predication. It is important to contrast the two methods of segmentation here. On the one hand, SALT relies heavily on intonation and pause criteria, and Loban only on grammatical decision rules, independent of pause or intonation criteria. One assumes that pause and intonation, however, go along with grammatical segmentation for the speaker.

Table 1
Segmentation Differences Between Loban and SALT
(Developed by Lena Caesar, Madison Metropolitan School District)

SALT	Loban
1. Then we gotta go home for supper and then I have another four "H" meeting until about eight o'clock.	1. Then we gotta go home for supper/ 2. And then I have another 4'H' meeting until . . . . /
2. It's a club for kids that want to be able to get into projects and take them to the fair.	3. It's a club for kids that want to be able to get into projects/ 4. And take them to the fair/
3. And I'll probably be sewing some stuff for 4H and I'll be take/ing my cat to the fair.	5. And I'll probably be taking some stuff for four H/ 6. And I'll be take/ing my cat to the fair/
4. And learn about things.	7. And learn about things/
5. And my meeting that I'm going to is with cross stitching.	8. And my meeting that I'm going to is with cross stitching/

* Adapted from *Language Development: Kindergarten through Grade Twelve*, by Walter Loban. © 1976. Urbana, IL: National Council of Teachers of English (NCTE). Used with permission.

Table 1 provides a comparison of segmentation decisions between SALT and Loban. It should be noted that either set of decisions can be used in performing analyses, including SALT analysis. When Loban criteria for segmentation are used, however, then the data to then interpret those analyses must be Loban's data and not the Reference Database data which uses SALT segmentation criteria.

II. Key concepts for this analysis

1. Communication units are independent clauses and their modifiers.
    A. Independent clause: a complete sentence that usually has a noun + verb in a subject-predicate relationship.
       1. Subjects generally indicate the topic of an utterance.
       2. Predicates which are verb phrases make comment(s) about the subject.
          example: The little boy went to school today.
                            (s)   (vp)
                   I drove the car.
                   (s) (vp)
    B. Dependent clause: part of the independent or main clause; typically cannot stand alone; joins with independent clause to add complexity and information; has a subject + verb, serves as noun, adjective, or adverb in the independent clause.
          example: The boy [who my father knows] went home.
                                (dependent clause)
2. Clause structure are compound clauses.
    A. Also known as compound clauses which are structurally complete and could stand as separate sentences (two independent clauses)
       1. Coordinating conjunctions to include: and, but, for, or, nor, yet
          example: I was hungry [but could not find a restaurant].
       2. Conjunctive adverbs to include: however, moreover, consequently
          example: The children wanted to play outside, [however it was raining].
    B. Dependent clause modifies the main clause and cannot stand alone
       1. Subordinating conjunctions to include: because, so, if, since, when, although
          example: [If you finish], you may go to the park.
       2. Relative pronouns to include: who, which, what, that
          example: I wonder [who she called].

III. The Analysis

The first step in the analysis is to identify the relevant units in the transcript. The major unit of this analysis is the communication unit (CU). CU's are defined as independent clauses and their relevant modifiers. Coordinating conjunctions and conjunctive adverbs separate a sentence into two independent clauses, two CU's. Subordinating conjunctions and relative pronouns divide a sentence into an independent and a dependent clause (modifier), which together represent one CU. The dependent clause is the second unit of analysis, documenting sentence complexity. The third unit is the maze: false starts, repetitions, and reformulations. Mazes are an index of word and utterance formulation fluency. These units and the number of words in these units will be used to calculate four measures: CU length, mean dependent clauses per CU, mean words per maze, and proportion of words in mazes as a percentage of total words.

1. Identifying CUs: The following examples will clarify the identification of CUs. Communication units are marked by (/)

> Example 1: and his mother says "now don't be ridiculous / you know you're eating an orange / and how can you starve to death while you're eating an orange?" / (3 units)

> Example 2: and so Johnny said "well if I weren't may I go down to the lollipop store?" / and she said "no, you've been down to the lollipop store too many times this week." / (2 units)

2. Mazes are confusions or tangles of words and/or word parts that occur while children are attempting to formulate messages. Mazes include the following:
   a. false starts
   b. repetitions
   c. reformulations
   d. abandoned/unfinished attempts

Mazes should be marked by (parentheses) to identify them for analysis.
> Example 1: (I'm going) I'm going to build a flying saucer.

> Example 2: I saw (a man) a hunter program last Sunday / (and he) and snow time he had to have lot (wah-h) when he got too many dogs, (he) and that's all I think of that picture./

3. Dependent clauses: Identify and place [brackets] around all dependent clauses. These have a subject and a verb and serve as a noun, adjective, or adverb in the independent clause. As noted earlier, they are introduced with subordinating conjunctions or relative pronouns which may be present or understood.

Following is a portion of a transcript that has been marked according to the above procedures.

> I think [this man went out just to have fun sailing one day] / and all of the sudden a storm came up, / and it looks [like he had a sail] / but it broke off./ There's also a tornado, I guess, (coming) coming at him from behind / and I think [he will signal to this ship in front of him and get help] /

IV. Computations

1. Average number of words per communication unit: CU Length

Count the total number of words in the narrative (after mazes have been removed) and divide by the number of communication units. Contractions are considered to be multiple words, e.g., "isn't" is two words, "s'a" (it is a) is three words. "Ain't" is counted as a single word. Each part of a name is a separate word, e.g., "John Smith" is two words. Simple infinitives such as "gonna" are two words. Refer to the data in Section 5 for score interpretation. Compare result to Loban's data in Table 2.

$$\frac{\text{Total Number of Words}}{\text{Total Number of Communication Unit}}$$

Table 2
Average Number of Words Per Communication Unit—Oral Language

Grade	Average Number of Words per Communication Unit (mean)			Relative Growth[a] (in percent)			Year-to-Year Velocity[b] (in percent)		
	High Group	Random Group	Low Group	High Group	Random Group	Low Group	High Group	Random Group	Low Group
1	7.91	6.88	5.91	67.61	58.80	50.51	----	----	----
2	8.10	7.56	6.65	69.23	64.62	56.84	+1.62	+ 5.82	+6.33
3	8.38	7.62	7.08	71.62	65.13	60.51	+2.39	+ 0.51	+3.67
4	9.28	9.00	7.55	79.32	76.92	64.53	+7.70	+ 11.79	+4.02
5	9.59	8.82	7.90	81.97	75.38	67.52	+2.65	− 1.54	+2.99
6	10.32	9.82	8.57	88.21	83.93	73.25	+6.24	+ 8.55	+5.73
7	11.14	9.75	9.01	95.21	83.33	77.01	+7.00	− 0.60	+3.76
8	11.59	10.71	9.52	99.06	91.54	81.37	+3.85	+ 8.21	+4.36
9	11.73	10.96	9.26	100.26	93.68	79.15	+1.20	+ 2.14	+2.22
10	12.34	10.68	9.41	105.47	91.28	80.43	+5.21	− 2.40	+1.28
11	13.00	11.17	10.18	111.11	95.47	87.01	+5.64	+ 4.19	+6.58
12	12.84	11.70	10.65	109.74	100.00	91.03	−1.37	+ 4.53	+4.02

2. Number of dependent clauses per communication unit: Structural Complexity

Count the number of dependent clauses and divide by the total number of communication units. Compare this score to the data in Table 3.

$$\frac{\text{Total Number of Dependent Clauses}}{\text{Number of Communication Units}}$$

Table 3
Average Number of Dependent Clauses Per Communication Unit—Oral Language

Grade	Average Number of Dependent Clauses per Unit (mean)			Relative Growth[a] (in percent)			Year-to-Year Velocity[b] (in percent)		
	High Group	Random Group	Low Group	High Group	Random Group	Low Group	High Group	Random Group	Low Group
1	0.24	0.16	0.12	41.38	27.59	20.69	----	----	----
2	0.25	0.21	0.17	43.10	36.21	29.31	+ 1.72	+ 8.62	+ 8.62
3	0.27	0.22	0.18	46.55	37.93	31.03	+ 3.45	+ 1.72	+ 1.72
4	0.37	0.30	0.20	63.79	51.72	34.48	+17.24	+ 13.79	+ 3.45
5	0.37	0.29	0.25	63.79	50.00	43.10	0.00	− 1.72	+ 8.62
6	0.41	0.37	0.30	70.69	63.79	51.72	+ 6.90	+ 13.79	+ 8.62
7	0.44	0.35	0.31	75.86	60.34	53.45	+ 5.17	− 3.45	+ 1.73
8	0.45	0.39	0.30	77.59	67.24	51.72	+ 1.73	+ 6.90	− 1.73
9	0.52	0.43	0.31	89.66	74.14	53.45	+12.07	+ 6.90	+ 1.73
10	0.61	0.48	0.33	105.17	82.76	56.90	+15.51	+ 8.62	+ 3.45
11	0.63	0.52	0.36	108.62	89.66	62.07	+ 3.45	+ 6.90	+ 5.17
12	0.67	0.58	0.46	115.52	100.00	79.31	+ 6.90	+ 10.34	+17.24

a Relative Growth uses the Random Group at grade twelve to equal 100 percent.
b Year-to-Year Velocity is the percentage change in any given group from one year to the following year.

3. Average number of words per maze: Maze Length

The average number of words per maze is the subject's total number of maze words divided by the number of mazes. A total of 20 maze words and 10 mazes would produce an average maze length of 20 words per maze. Compare this score to the data in Table 4.

$$\frac{\text{Number of Maze Words}}{\text{Number of Mazes}} = \text{Average Maze Length}$$

Table 4
Average Number of Words Per Maze—Oral Language
(mean)

Grade	High Group	Random Group	Low Group
1	1.94	2.09	1.81
2	1.89	1.89	1.90
3	1.88	1.85	1.98
4	1.97	2.06	1.99
5	1.93	2.09	2.07
6	2.15	2.21	2.16
7	1.90	2.06	2.17
8	1.96	2.01	2.11
9	1.78	1.98	2.18
10	1.85	1.92	1.92
11	1.94	1.97	1.97
12	1.77	1.99	2.24

4. Maze words as a percentage of total words: Maze Density

The number of words in mazes is a simple index of the child's fluency in formulating utterances. If the child produces 450 words in communication units and 50 words in mazes, for a total of 500 words, the ratio would be 50:500 or 10 percent of all verbal productions. Compare this score to the data in Table 5.

$$\frac{\text{Number of Maze Words}}{\text{Total Number of Words}}$$

Table 5

Maze Words as a Percentage of Total Words—Oral Language

Grade	High Group	Random Group	Low Group
1	7.61	7.46	9.04
2	6.21	8.03	8.31
3	4.71	6.39	7.98
4	6.39	8.38	11.06
5	6.41	7.53	9.04
6	6.98	8.29	10.33
7	5.82	7.76	11.08
8	6.08	8.12	9.30
9	5.31	7.29	10.18
10	7.45	7.40	7.51
11	7.32	7.04	9.01
12	7.25	7.04	9.19

Comparison Sample

The Oakland, California children whose data are summarized in Table 3 were studied for 13 years. The low group constituted the bottom 16 percent of the total group in terms of cumulative teacher ratings of oral language ability (median IQ = 88); the high group, the top 16 percent (median IQ = 116); and the random group, a sample representative of the full SES spectrum in Oakland (median IQ = 100). They were selected from a larger group of 211; each group in the tables has 35 children in it. The three groups are all of diverse ethnic makeup but differ in socioeconomic status: children in the high group come predominately from families with skilled occupations; those in the low group, from families with unskilled occupations.

Example Loban Analysis

Client: _____ Date: _____

Clinician: _____ Amount of time: _____

Narrative topic(s): _____

_____

_____

Directions: Number each of your communication units. In segmenting the transcript, use / to set off communication units, ( ) for mazes, and [ ] for dependent clauses.

		# of Words	# of Dependent Clauses	Mazes	# of Maze Words
1.	(Webb's, his) his name is Webb	4	0	1	2
2.	And he's a little funny guy.	7	0		
3.	And he's real funny, super funny.	7	0		
4.	And . . . on the one show he said "are you XXX?"	9	0		1
5.	He says "are you (StuartXX) Mr. Cully?"	6	0	1	
6.	He's super funny.	4	0		
7.	(And she's . . .) You know what?	3	0	1	2
8.	(He's . . . the . . .) you know he told (his girlfriend, I mean) his friend [that (um he, he) one time, he ran away].	11	1	3	11
9.	"Cause (his mama was having) his mom and dad were having a fight / (an) and . . . . "	9	0	2	5
10.	Webb was telling . . . his friend.	6	0		
11.	and (. . . the) the guy said "OK, I'll run away."	9	0	1	1
12.	(So . . .) and the guy says "Why I doesn't say you had to."	12	0	1	1
13.	(Webb says um and then so) he says "I think [I'll go to Miami]."	9	1	1	6
14.	And then she . . . leaves.	4	0		
15.	And she goes packing, [while she's at Webb's house].	10	1		
16.	And mom doesn't know [that she's there].	9	1		
17.	(Goes) stays there and has cup of coffee.	7	0	1	1
18.	And Webb comes down.	4	0		
19.	"Hey, where's your friend?"	5	0		
20.	(He says . . . . In m . . . I mean) in Miami XX he says	4	0	1	5
21.	Where'd he go?	4	0		
22.	And he goes back up in his room and says	10	0		

		# of Words	# of Dependent Clauses	Mazes	# of Maze Words
23.	He starts praying at his (um) bed, you know.	8	0	1	1
24.	And she's under the bed.	6	0		
25.	And then the (mom) dad walks in, Webb's dad.	8	0	1	1
26.	Says "where's your friends?"	5	0		
27.	The girl crawls under the bed.	6	0		
28.	"How you doing there?"	4	0		
29.	"I'm back."	3	0		
30.	(Says . . .) An' Webb says, "How come you're back so quick?"	10	0	1	1
Total:		**203**	**4**	**16**	**39**

Average number words/CU: 6.77
Average number dependent clauses/CU: 0.13
Percentage of CU's with mazes: 46%
Average maze length: 2.78

Resources

The following list of publications has been compiled to provide further information about complex language analyses that are beyond the scope of this guide. The list is divided into several sections beginning with general sources covering LSA from a variety of perspectives. These references have been selected to provide a broad coverage of LSA on the one hand and the best materials for further reading on narrative analysis and linguistically and culturally diverse populations on the other. These lists are not intended to be exhaustive, but provide a starting point for further reading. The trend in the development of LSA strategies was initially driven by a focus on syntax which has given way to a focus on broader pragmatic issues, particularly narrative structure. The authors expect that advances in narrative analysis will complement the general analyses presented in this guide and ultimately provide links to the acquisition of literacy skills. Speech and language experts are just beginning to realize the power of LSA to inform educators about the linguistic knowledge and adaptive strategies children employ in communication.

Note: In Appendix H, tables documenting specific linguistic differences in Black English, Hispanic English, and Asian English can be found.

General Books:

Brinton, B. and M. Fujiki. *Conversational Management with Language Impaired Children*. Rockville, MD: Aspen Publishers Inc., 1989.

Crystal, D. *Profiling Language Disability*. London: Edward Arnold Pub., Inc., 1982.

Crystal, D., ed. *Working with LARSP*. New York: Elsiver, 1979.

Gallagher, T., ed. *Pragmatics of Language: Clinical Practice Issues*. San Diego, CA: Singular Publishing Group, 1991.

Larson, V. and N. McKinley. *Communication Assessment and Intervention Strategies for Adolescents*. Eau Claire, WI: Thinking Publications, 1987.

Lund, N. and J. Duchan. *Assessing Children's Language in Naturalistic Contexts: 2nd edition*. Englewood Cliffs, NJ: Prentice-Hall, Inc., 1988.

McTear, M. *Children's Conversation*. Oxford, England: Basil Blackwell Co., 1985.

Retherford-Stickler, K. *Guide to Analysis of Language Transcripts*. Eau Claire, WI: Thinking Publications, 1987.

Simon, C. *Communication Skills and Classroom Success: Assessment and Therapy Methodologies for Language and Learning Disabled Students*. Eau Claire, WI: Thinking Publications, 1991.

Wallach, G. and L. Miller. *Language Intervention and Academic Success*. Boston, MA: College Hill Press, 1988.

Wisconsin Administrative Code, Chapter 11, Wisconsin Department of Public Instruction.

Pragmatic and Discourse Analysis:

Liles, B. "Cohesion in the Narratives of Normal and Language Disordered Children." *Journal of Speech and Hearing Research.* 28 (1985), pp. 123-133.

Merritt, D. and B. Liles. "Narrative Analysis: Clinical Applications of Story Generation and Story Re-telling." *Journal of Speech and Hearing Disorders* 54.3 (1989), pp. 438-447.

Norris, J. and R. Bruning. "Cohesion in the Narratives of Good and Poor Readers." *Journal of Speech and Hearing Disorders* 53 (1988), pp. 416-424.

Prutting, C. and D. Kirchner. "A Clinical Appraisal of the Pragmatic Aspects of Language." *Journal of Speech and Hearing Disorders* 52.2 (1987), pp. 105-119.

Scott, C. "A Perspective on the Evaluation of School Children's Narratives." *Language Speech and Hearing Services in Schools* 19 (1988), pp. 67-82.

Resource Recommendations for LCD Populations In Wisconsin

Section 1: General Information

Brinton, D., M. Snow, and M. Wesche. *Content-based Second Language Acquisition.* New York: Newbury House Publishers, 1989.

Cummins, J. *Bilingualism and Special Education: Issues in Assessment and Pedagogy.* San Diego, CA: College Hill Press, 1984.

Fradd, S. and W. Tikunoff. *Bilingual Education and Bilingual Special Education: A Guide for Administrators.* San Diego, CA: Singular Publishing Group Inc., 1987.

McLaughlin, B. *Second Language Acquisition in Childhood - Volume 2: School Aged Children.* Hillsdale, NJ: LEA, 1985.

Miller, N. *Bilingualism and Language Disability: Assessment and Remediation.* San Diego, CA: College Hill Press, 1984.

Padilla, A., H. Fairchild, and C. Valadez. *Bilingual Education Issues and Strategies.* Newbury Park, CA: Sage Publications, 1990.

Skutnabb-Kangas, T. and J. Cummins. *Minority Education: From Shame to Struggle.* Philadelphia: Multilingual Matters, 1988.

Section 2: Specific Population Information

African-American:

Benson-Hale, J. *Black Children: Their Roots, Culture and Learning Style.* Revised edition. Baltimore, MD: Johns Hopkins University Press, 1986.

Cole, Lorraine. *Resource Guide to Multicultural Tests and Materials in Communicative Disorders.* Rockville, MD: ASHA Publications, 1987.

Edwards, J. *Language Advantage and Disadvantage.* San Diego, CA: Singular Publishing Group Inc., 1989.

Taylor, O. *Nature of Communication Disorders in Culturally and Linguistically Diverse Populations.* San Diego, CA: Singular Publishing Group Inc., 1986.

Taylor, O. *Treatment of Communication Disorders in Culturally and Linguistically Diverse Populations.* San Diego, CA: Singular Publishing Group Inc., 1986.

Wolfram, W. *Dialects and American English.* Englewood Cliffs, NJ: Prentice-Hall, 1990.

American Indian:

Johnson, M. J. and B. A. Ramirez. *American Indian Exceptional Children and Youth.* Reston, VA: Council for Exceptional Children, 1987.

Reyhner, J. *Language Education Practices and Native Language Survival.* Billings, MT: Eastern Montana College, 1990.

Reyhner, J. *Teaching the Indian Child.* 2nd edition. Billings, MT: Eastern Montana College, 1988.

Wisconsin Woodland Project: Rhinelander, Wisconsin
information relative to: American Indian history, American Indian tribes in Wisconsin, American Indian/Anglo-American relations, American Indian culture (1-800-293-8932).

Asian: Hmong

Bliatout, B. T., et al. *Handbook for Teaching Hmong-Speaking Students.* Folsom, CA: Folsom Cordova Unified School District. Southeast Asia Community Resource Center, 1988.

Cheng, L. *Assessing Asian Language Performance: Guidelines for Evaluating Limited English Proficient Students.* Rockville, MD: Aspen Publishers Inc., 1987.

Hmoob Lub Neej Tshiab Nyob Hauv Ameslikas / New Hmong Life in America. Videotape. Worthwhile Films, 104 King Street, Madison, WI 53703, (608) 251-8855. $30.00.

McGinn, F. and J. McMenamin. *Acquiring English: An ESL Teacher's Guide for the Hmong Student.* Los Angeles, CA: Evaluation Dissemination and Assessment Center, California State University, 1984.

McInnis, K. M., H. E. Patracchi, and M. Morgenbesser. *The Hmong in America: Providing Ethnic-Sensitive Health, Education, and Human Services.* Dubuque, IA: Kendall/Hunt Publishing Co., 1990.

Roop, P. and C. Roop. *The Hmong In America: We Sought Refuge Here.* Appleton, WI: Appleton Area School District, 1990.

Trueba, H. T., L. Jacobs, and E. Kirton. *Cultural Conflict and Adaptation*. New York: The Falmer Press, 1990.

Hispanic

Ortiz, A. and B. Ramirez. *Schools and the Culturally Diverse Exceptional Student: Promising Practices and Future Directions*. Reston, VA: Council for Exceptional Children, 1988.

See also chapters in Skutnabb-Kangas and Cummins (1988) and Taylor (1986), listed above.

Section 3: *Journal Recommendations for LCD Populations*

Language, Speech and Hearing Services in the Schools
Journal of Speech and Hearing Disorders
Journal of Speech and Hearing Research
American Speech and Hearing Association (ASHA)
10801 Rockville Pike
Rockville, MD 20852-3279

Exceptional Children
Council for Exceptional Children
1920 Association Avenue
Reston, VA 22091

Journal of Reading
International Reading Association
800 Barksdale Road
P. O. Box 8139
Newark, DE 19714
(302) 731-1600

TESOL Quarterly
Georgetown University
Suite 205
1118 22nd Street, N. W.
Washington, DC 20037

Topics in Language Disorders
Aspen Publishers Inc.
1600 Research Blvd.
Rockville, MD 20850
(301)-251-8500

Section 4: *Agencies to contact for additional information*

American Speech and Hearing Association (ASHA)
Office of Minority Affairs
Attn: Vicki Deal
10801 Rockville Pike
Rockville, MD 20852-3279
(301) 897-5700

National Indian Education Clearinghouse
Arizona State University
Tempe, AZ
(602)-965-6490

Southeast Asian Refugee Studies Project/Newsletter
University of Minnesota
330 Hubert H. Humphrey Center
301 19th Avenue S.
Minneapolis, MN 55455

Glossary

Assigning Structure Stage: Detailed descriptive procedure for the analysis of syntactic development for the following structures; 14 grammatical morphemes, noun and verb phrase elaboration, negation, WH and yes/no questions, and complex sentences.

Asynchronies: rate of development which is not simultaneous either between language comprehension and language production or among language levels (vocabulary, syntax, or semantics) within comprehension or production.

Auxiliary verb: accompanies a main verb, for example, is, are, was were, do, have. He *is* running, or They *were* running.

CALSA: *Computer Assisted Language Sample Analysis*

CAP: An analysis of social assertiveness of child speech designed by Marc Fey. See the resource section, Appendix D, for the reference to Fey's book which details the analysis procedure.

CHILDES: *Child Language Data Exchange System.* Developed to provide researchers and clinicians access to transcripts of child language collected for a variety of developmental studies. The CHILDES system includes hundreds of transcripts dating from Roger Brown's Adam, Eve and Sarah, to recent transcripts from a variety of child and adult populations. The system has developed a number of computer analyses routines that run on IBM and Macintosh computers.

Circumlocution: An avoidance behavior involving word selection of utterance formulation choices avoiding difficult areas in constructing messages. The result usually fails to communicate clearly. These utterances can be diagnostic of word finding or utterance formulation deficits.

Cognitive abilities: Mental abilities applied to experience or knowledge and demonstrated by skills such as classification, sequencing, and memory.

Cognitively disabled: Recently adopted term replacing mental retardation.

Computerized Profiling: A set of computer programs designed to perform a series of grammatical, semantic, and pragmatic analyses from coded transcripts of child speech.

Contingent speech: utterance(s)/sentence(s) that are obligated by the preceding utterance or question and usually continue the topic, provide answers, add information, question, modify, or repeat information.

Conversational partner: any person sharing a conversation. Usually used to refer to the adult role in conversing with a child.

CU: Content Unclear. A code used to mark utterances where the meaning cannot be determined by the listener (transcriber). This may occur for the individual utterance as a message unit or where the utterance content is unclear relative to the contingency specified by the preceding utterance.

Dichotomy: Division into two parts or classes, for example, the language characteristics that allow SLPs to distinguish between difference versus disorder or disorder versus normal performance.

Elicitation: Refers to the process of directing the child to produce utterances of a specific type, containing specific content or within a specified speaking context like narration.

EU: Error at the utterance level. A code used to note an error involving phrase or clause level units or the entire utterance usually coded at the time of transcription.

EW: Error at the word level. A code used to note word level errors usually coded at the time of transcription.

False start: When a speaker starts an utterance or utterance segment, stops, and returns to its starting point and attempts the word or utterance segment again. For example, "Th, The boy went . . . . "

Formulation load: Used here to describe the difficulty confronting the speaker when trying to communicate messages in different situations. The difficulty speakers face in situations where they must remember all of the referents, relations, and temporal sequence versus situations where listeners contribute equally, as in conversation and narration.

Grammatical functors: Words that support the semantic context, such as articles, pronouns, conjunctions, and auxiliary verbs but do not express the major semantic roles of agent, action, adverbial, etc.

Intonation contour: The melodic pattern of the utterance. Used here to refer to utterance segmentation criteria involving the rising intonation of questions or falling intonation marking the end of utterances that are statements or comments.

LARSP: *Language Assessment, Remediation and Screening Procedure*, a detailed procedure for the analysis of syntax.

Language Sample Analysis: A procedure based on the recording and transcription of a sample of dialogue providing opportunity for the analysis of language production in the areas of syntax, semantics, and pragmatic, in a variety of speaking conditions.

LCD: Linguistically and culturally diverse. Used to designate persons learning English as a second language or from various ethnic or cultural groups.

LEP: Limited English Proficiency. Used to refer to children from culturally and linguistically diverse backgrounds, learning English as a second language.

Lexical: Refers to the word or vocabulary level of analysis. Lexicon refers to the total vocabulary available to an individual child.

Lingquest I: A computer program for Apple II computers that performs a grammatical analysis on a coded transcript of child speech.

Linguistic: Referring to the formal properties of a language, the syntax, lexicon (vocabulary), semantic, or discourse features.

Loban: Walter Loban who developed a procedure for the analysis of oral language skill in school age children.

Loban Analysis: A set of analysis performed on 30 narrative utterances documenting utterance length, complexity and maze frequency, and density. Norms are provided by grade level, K-12. See Appendix C for a summary.

Marking Bound Morphemes: Coding bound morphemes using a "/" to identify them for computer analysis as in possession (/z), plural (/s), past tense (/ed), and third person singular verb (/3s).

Maze: A set of behaviors identified by Loban including false starts, repetitions, and reformulations of words, parts of words, or phrases noting difficulty in formulating words or utterances. Mazes are coded in transcripts using parentheses ( ) to be able to analyze them as well as exclude them from the main body of the utterance.

Metalinguistic: The ability to consciously think about, talk about, judge, correct, and explain language and its properties.

MLU: Mean (average) Length of Utterance, a general measure of syntactic development in production. As utterances get longer, they generally get more complex structurally. Usually calculated in morphemes, the minimal meaningful unit in a language.

Modal: A verb which indicates speaker attitude/mood and accompanies the main verb, for example, wish/ intention (will, shall), possibility/certainty (can, could, may, might), and obligation/necessity (must, should).

Morphemes: The minimal unit of meaning of a language. Usually defined as a word root, a prefix, or a suffix. The word "boy" is one morpheme, the word "boy/s" is two morphemes.

Morphology: The rule system governing words as units and the rules for combining free (root words) with bound morphemes (prefixes, suffixes, etc.).

Narrative: A story or other type of discourse characterized minimally by events linked by temporal (time) and/or causal relationships.

NDW: Number of different words. A measure of semantic diversity. One of the measures of developmental progress, significantly correlating with chronological age in the reference database data set.

Oblique: An obscure, indirect, or not obvious reference.

156

Omissions: word(s) or bound morpheme(s) that are not produced but should have been included in an utterance. Marked by an asterisk (*) in the transcript to note something was omitted.

On-line transcription: Transcription of a language sample as it is taking place.

Orthogonal: Intersecting or lying at right angles, or having perpendicular slopes or tangents at the point of intersection. Used here to refer to the relationship among variables, as MLU increases, chronological age increases as well.

Orthography: The representation of the sounds of a language by written or printed symbols.

Overlaps: simultaneous speaking by two speakers, marked by enclosing the segments in arrows (< >).

PAL: *Pye Analysis of Language*. A series of computer assisted language analyses designed by Cliff Pye at the University of Kansas.

PALSA: *Parrot Easy Language Sample Analysis*. A computer program design to perform simple analysis on a sample of child speech.

Phonology: study of the sound system of a language and the rules for combining sounds to form words.

Pragmatic: The study of how a speaker uses the language system in a variety of social environments, with various participants, for a variety of purposes.

Pre-set analysis: A feature of SALT where analyses are pre-configured and available to the user by menu selection.

PRISM: Two analyses of vocabulary designed by David Crystal to inventory lexical diversity by category, and the grammatical categorization of the lexicon.

Propositional embedding: one type of subordination used in semantic analysis; utterance unit that functions as the object or participant of the main utterance unit (Bill thought *he would wash the car*).

Prosody: melody, tone, or rhythmic characteristics used in language to signal word and sentence meaning.

Psychometric: The study of test development and construction involving establishing the reliability and validity of a measure; establishing norms on an appropriately stratified sample of the population.

RDB: Reference database. A database found in Appendix A containing a summary of the language sample analysis results from 266 Wisconsin children in conversation and narrative speaking conditions.

Reformulation: An utterance correction where the speaker begins an utterance, then begins again changing a word, part word, or phrase. Included as one type of maze in both the SALT and Loban analyses.

Responses: Generally refers to answers to questions or other utterances obligating the listener to respond.

SALT: *Systematic Analysis of Language Transcripts*. A computer program designed to analyze language production between two speakers.

Segmentation: The process of dividing the acoustic stream of speech into words and utterances in the transcription process.

Semantics: The study of meaning expressed in language through words and sentences.

Semi-auxiliaries: early modal verb forms, such as wanna, hafta, gonna, gotta, sposta.

SLP: Speech Language Pathologist

Speech motor maturation: The development and coordination of the respiratory, phonatory, and articulatory systems as related to speech rate, intelligibility, and language production.

Synchronous: rate of development which occurs simultaneously within language levels, vocabulary, syntax, semantics, and across language processes, comprehension, and production.

Syntax: The study of the grammatical rules of a language.

Timing: 1) Refers to a series of analyses related to speaking rate or pausing. 2) The duration of a transcript expressed in minutes and seconds. 3) Final (total) time coded in clock or military time and marked with a hyphen (-13:04; -12:15) at the end of a SALT transcript allowing timing variable to be calculated.

Timing markers: 1) Minute markers noted with a hyphen (-); coded in clock or military time (-1:00; -2:00). 2) Pauses may be marked and timing noted within utterances or between utterances.

TNW: Total number of words. Refers to a measure of verbal fluency or proficiency when words are counted in a transcript of a specific duration, for example, 12 minutes. TNW is one of the measures of developmental progress significantly correlating with chronological age in the reference database data set.

Transcription: The process of representing spoken language in written form using standard English orthography or IPA.

Transcription conventions: Conventions using symbols, codes, or spellings to mark various features on a language transcript.

Type token ratio (TTR): Ratio between number of different words to total number words in 50 utterances used as an indicator of semantic diversity.

Typology: The unique types of language production disorders including sentence formulation, word finding, rate, discourse/pragmatic, semantic/reference, and delay.

User-specified analysis: A SALT analysis feature where the user can specify the units of language to be analyzed, coded, or counted.

Utterance segmentation: The process of identifying utterances using intonation pattern (rising or falling pitch contour) and pause time boundaries.

Cost Effectiveness

Although the greatest benefit of Language Sample Analysis is the improved service to Wisconsin students, LSA addresses other practical issues as well. Administrators will be happy to note that LSA is highly cost-effective in two specific areas: transcription and computer-aided analysis.

Transcription

One of the barriers to using LSA until this time has been the significant amount of SLP time required to transcribe the language sample. SLPs with high caseloads simply did not have the uninterrupted time to complete this aspect of the process. Therefore, as a result of a grant funded by the Department of Public Instruction, several transcription laboratories have already been developed (CESA 9, CESA 8, Milwaukee Public Schools) and several other areas are expecting to establish them in the near future. The prototype for these laboratories was developed by the Madison Metropolitan School District with the support of Dr. Jon Miller and the computing facility at the University of Wisconsin-Madison Waisman Center. These transcription laboratories have trained clerical personnel in the transcription process making it more cost effective. In addition, the transcription laboratories have SALT and SALT Profiles available to provide computer-assisted analysis of the language samples after they are transcribed.

Using one of these laboratories or establishing a transcription laboratory of one's own (if a large district) is an administrative solution that can free SLPs for the more difficult tasks of interpretation of the data obtained from the child's language sample rather than bogging them down with the time-consuming and mechanical process of transcription. The focus provided by a transcription laboratory will allow both SLPs and transcribers to hone their skills and produce better, more accurate, and less time-consuming analyses.

Computer-aided Analysis

It is clear that computers offer a number of significant advantages over doing LSA by hand. While there will be some initial additional purchase of software, training of staff, and purchase of computers (if not already available within the district); computer-assisted LSA is cost-efficient in the long run. The professional time saved both in terms of assessment and planning of appropriate intervention strategies (makes computer-aided LSA very cost effective). Another cost benefit comes as a result of being able to reduce the number of students who are placed inappropriately in speech and language programs. Due to the more in-depth analysis provided by LSA, these inappropriate placements and resultant costs are reduced.

In anticipating costs associated with implementing computer-assisted LSA, consideration should be given to the following factors: hardware, software, staff training. Specific costs can be obtained by contacting the RSN Director of CESA 9, or Dr. Jon Miller, Waisman Center, University of Wisconsin-Madison.

School districts may wish to work cooperatively in implementing a computer-assisted laboratory or transcription service for language sample analysis, or contact the already established transcription laboratories to purchase some service time. In the long run, the cost effectiveness of computer solutions to LSA will be demonstrated by

- the breadth and depth of the diagnostic data they provide;
- improved definitions of language impairment;
- databased decisions regarding whether the child has an EEN; and
- more effective and efficient intervention programs.

Sample Case Studies

Case One: Utterance Formulation Problems
Chronological Age (CA): 10-7, Grade 4
Features of the Utterance Formulation Category
- maze revisions at word and phrase level units,
- increased mean length of utterance,
- pauses within and between utterances, and
- word order errors.

Background Information/Reason for Referral
This child was referred because of difficulty in all aspects of language arts: reading, writing, and processing information presented auditorily in the context of her fourth grade classroom. She is viewed as socially competent and polite and interacts appropriately with both adults and peers. Three of her older siblings are identified as handicapped in the areas of learning disabilities and speech and language. This student uses both Standard Black English and Standard American English dialects.

Results of Standardized Testing

Peabody Picture Vocabulary Test—Revised:
Standard Score (SS) 88
22 percentile

Expressive One Word Picture Vocabulary Test:
Standard Score (SS) 88
21 percentile

Test of Language Development—Intermediate:

Characteristics	SS 6	9 percentile
Grammatical Comprehension	SS 6	9 percentile
Generals	SS 7	16 percentile
Sentence Combining	SS 3	1 percentile
Word Ordering	SS 3	1 percentile

Weschler Intelligence Scale for Children—Revised: (WISC-R)
Verbal 69
Performance 102
Full Scale 60-84

Kaufman Assessment Battery for Children:
Sequential Processing 93
Simultaneous Processing 85

Academic testing confirmed significant difficulty with reading and writing. Math performance was at grade level.

Standardized test results suggest a significant delay in language comprehension and production with average non-verbal skills. She appears to be having the most difficulty in the area of syntax where her performance is significantly delayed. Her skills across measures of semantics are in the low average range.

Transcript of Conversational Language Sample

A conversational language sample was elicited and transcribed. The following is an excerpt from the transcript:

194 E That show we had yesterday in the gym was science, was/n't it?
195 C Mhm.
196 E Can you tell me something about what you saw?
197 C (H*) I saw like you know those (glow in or) light/s they like glow
198   in the dark.
199 C They snap/ed them and then they like twist/ed them up
200   straighten them out [EU].
201 C Well (whe) when I got on the bus, there was this one girl that
202   had the purple one that they snap/ed.
203 C (She did/n't she did/n't) they did/n't say take it (because they
204   would/n't give one) they would give everybody one, and she
205   stoled [EO:stole] it after the table [eu].
206 E She did?
207 C And she/'s in Miss (Ro* m*) Romereck/z class.
208 E I think she/'s in XX.
209 E Yeah she/'s in XX.
210 E I/'ve forgotten who it ws.
211 E Susie?
212 C Not Susie.
213 E No.
214 C (Sh* this girl was in, b*, girl with a, I think I) yeah she/'s in
215   there.
216 C She girl with a braid/s up in her hair, like has it over there and
217   always wear
218   (This p*) that pink coat.

Analysis of the Data

The language sample transcript was analyzed using SALT and the child's performance was compared to typically developing 11 year olds in the Reference Database. Significant data is summarized in the chart below. As one can see, she produced a higher number of mazes than the normal students. Almost 50 percent of her utterances, or more than three standard deviations above the mean, had mazes. Of the 77 mazes she produced, 40 were revisions. These revisions often resulted in pronoun or syntax changes which did not always help clarify or repair her message for the listener. Many utterances had multiple mazes which further interfered with effective communication. The total number of words and number of different words were more than one standard deviation above the mean. This reflects her strategy of talking a lot to be sure that her message is successfully understood before she moves on to another topic. It is also consistent with standardized test scores which suggested that she had approximately average ability in semantics.

Personal pronouns occurred more frequently (two standard deviations above the mean) in this language sample than in the samples collected from normal 11 year olds. She used pronouns instead of proper names. The listener is able to make assumptions about who she is referring to because of shared knowledge and other semantic clues provided in the course of the conversation.

Measurement Category	Student	Mean of Eleven Year Olds	Standard Deviation
Utterances with Mazes	57	24	10
TTR	.35	.43	.06
Number Total Words	1026	693	172
Number Different Words	288	229	38
Personal Pronouns			
Total	168	90	27
Type	12	10	1

Further analysis revealed numerous word level errors, usually the incorrect use of tense markers, and discourse level errors.

Intervention Plan

An intervention plan was designed to increase the specificity of her language. She works on reducing the number of pronouns she uses rather than proper names and specific nouns. The content of the classroom is used as a strategy to implement this goal. As a result, she practices the vocabulary, concepts, and content needed for academics and reduces the number of mazes in her utterances since she no longer needs to revise her pronoun choices. In addition, she is encouraged to make specific "lists" (for example, tell me everything you know about . . .). She and her clinician then combine the lists into complex sentence patterns. The practice of syntactic patterns is facilitating utterance formulation, which in turn results in fewer mazes.

Case Two: Rate Problem—Hyper-verbal
C.A.: 8, Grade 2
Features of the Rate—Hyper-verbal Category
• increased number of utterances and words per minute which may be combined with reduced semantic content.

Background Information/Reason for Referral

This child attended Head Start for two years prior to entering full day kindergarten. He received Chapter I assistance during kindergarten and first grade. A referral was made to exceptional education at the beginning of his second grade year because of continuing academic and language problems in spite of trying hard, having good work habits, and modified instructional strategies within regular education. He is a student who uses Standard American English dialect. Two siblings receive exceptional education in learning disabilities and speech and language.

Results of Standardized Testing

Test of Language Development—Primary:
Picture Vocabulary	SS 9
Oral Vocabulary	SS 8
Grammatic Completion	SS 8
Grammatic Understanding	SS 9

Peabody Picture Vocabulary Test—R:
SS 77

Expressive One Word Picture Vocabulary Test:
SS 81

Token Test, Part V:
within normal limits

WISC—R:
V 108
P 84
FS 96

Reading and written language skills were assessed to be at least 50 percent discrepant from expected achievement. Math performance was at grade level.

The standardized testing information suggests a profile of a student who has overall average potential, and relative strengths in verbal skills. Specific language skills are in the low average range with more difficulty in receptive vocabulary. This student's classroom teacher did not feel that the test scores adequately reflected the difficulties the child was having using and understanding language in the classroom.

Transcript of a Conversational Language Sample

A conversational language sample was elicited and transcribed. The following is an excerpt from the transcript:

36		E	Tell me about it.
37		C	See when I crack/ed the egg open I had to take the yolk of out of
38			the egg and put it in the bowl.
39		C	And we did/n't make an egg, but I could/'ve made a [EW:an] egg out
40			of *it if I had a fork and a stove and a pot.
41	=	E	laughs
42		E	Uhhuh.
43		E	Then what did you do?
44		C	Then we had this little tube and at the end it was real big.
45		C	It had a cannon thing in it.
46		E	It had a what thing?
47		C	It was a big old machine we had.
48		C	We had to get some little piece/s that we made and we stuck it
49			[EW: them] on there [CU].
50		C	(Then) then we would pour the egg in it.
51		C	Then it/'s sposta blow up and it did.
52		E	It did?
53		C	Yeah but not fire smoke.
54		C	(Just) it just said pow!
55		C	But everybody had to stay away from it because I/'m the only one
56			who knew what I was do/ing.
57		E	(What blew) excuse me, what blew up?
58		C	The (um) whole egg and then (when) when we took it out it was a
59			whole egg.
60		C	It was cook/ed.
61		E	Really?
62		C	A fried egg, yeah.
63		E	Huh!
64		C	Then we gotta make it into a whole so enough for everybody to
65			have some.
66		C	And then (we had) all of us had our egg.
67		E	Were they hardboiled egg/s?

68   C They were fried egg/s.
69   E Tell me about the machine you put it in.
70   E I don't get that part.
71   C The machine (it was) it was a big old box that we made.
72   C We put the wire/s in.
73   C We just found the XX.
74   C We got alot of>
75   C (Me and Kenny) me and Kenny was the only one that know what
76   we was do/ing [EU].
77   C We got a whole bunch of piece/s.
78   C We build [EW:built] it up.
79   C Then we build [EW:built] that whole thing up at school.
80   C (We f*) we stay/ed in for a recess.
81   C We (took s*) got some wire/s that (I had broke up) I had to break
82   up.
83   C I bought a robot and broke it up.
84   C And then^
85   E You bought a what and broke it up?
86   C I brought a robot <> and then I smashed it.

Analysis of the Data

The conversational sample was analyzed using SALT and the results were compared to the typically developing seven and nine year olds in the reference database. The data is summarized in the chart below. Of particular note is the amount of talking produced by this child. Both utterance attempts per minute and words per minute measures were more than two standard deviations above the mean for students in the normal sample. His mean length of utterance was also elevated: more than three standard deviations above the mean for seven year olds and two standard deviations for nine year olds. At the same time, his TTR was three standard deviations below the mean for seven year olds and two standard deviations below the mean for nine year olds. Thus, although he talked a lot and in lengthy utterances, the content and semantic diversity of his conversation was limited.

Measurement Category	Student	Mean Seven Year Olds	Standard Deviation	Mean Nine Year Olds	Standard Deviation
Type Token Ratio	.30	.45	.05	.44	.06
Number Total Words	810	524	73	592	94
Number Different Words	226	188	17	209	26
MLU	8.10	5.76	.79	6.50	1.04
Number Personal Pronouns					
Total	139	80	14	85	16
Type	30	9	1	9	1
Mazes	30	26	12	25	8

The number of mazes in the sample was slightly high, but within one standard deviation of the mean for both seven and nine year olds. The mazes consisted mostly of repetitions of words and phrases which did not interfere with communication.

The printed transcript allowed the clinician to further describe how this student has difficulty fitting information into a logical and organized framework of knowledge that enables him to retrieve and express ideas easily. Very little functional information is related, and the sequence of events had little to do with what actually happened in his classroom. He has little regard for the difficulty his communication partner experiences following the content, and did not self-monitor or make repairs.

Intervention Plan

Language therapy for this student focuses on comprehension and production of semantics. The clinician coordinates therapy activities with classroom academic instruction in order to pre-teach and review specific vocabulary needed for academics. Words with multiple meanings and analogies are both therapy targets. In addition, classification and semantic mapping strategies were used to facilitate the organization of a logical mental framework. The student is encouraged to formulate thoughts and utterances before talking to reduce impulsivity and focus the content of his message.

Case Three: Rate Problem—Hypo-verbal
C.A.: 6-11, Grade 1
Features of the Rate—Hypo-verbal Category
- decreased number of utterances and words per minute
- pauses within and between utterances

Background Information/Reason for Referral

This child was referred to exceptional education by his first grade classroom teacher because of language and academic concerns. After screening, adjustments were made in his academic schedule to allow him to attend kindergarten for a portion of each morning. Private tutoring for academic skill reinforcement was also arranged by his family. These modifications in curriculum and instruction appeared to be adequate to support learning at an appropriate rate, however, concerns about language comprehension and production persisted.

Results of Standardized Testing

Test of Language Development—Primary:

Picture Vocabulary	SS 2	75 percentile
Oral Vocabulary	SS 7	16 percentile
Grammatical Understanding	SS 8	25 percentile
Grammatical Completion	SS 7	16 percentile
Sentence Imitation	SS 9	37 percentile
Word Articulation	SS 13	84 percentile
Word Discrimination	SS 10	50 percentile

Peabody Picture Vocabulary Test—R:
SS 100
50 percentile

Boehm Test of Basic Concepts:
37/50 correct
1 percentile

WISC—R:
V 95
P 91
FS 92

166

Comprehension of language, except when concepts were embedded into longer directions as on the *Boehm*, appeared to be within average limits. His classroom teacher reported that he did not appear to understand directions or lengthy and complex oral presentations. In contrast, language production subtests were delayed.

Transcript of a Conversational Language Sample

A conversational language sample was elicited and transcribed. The following is an excerpt from that sample:

65 E And you have a sister?
66 C Mhm.
67 E Named [p].
68 C Sandra.
69 E Oh, ok.
70 E What/'s your favorite thing to do with your family?
71 C (Um) eat.
72 E Yeah?
73 E Tell me some more about that.
74 C Eat Chinese food.
75 E Oh yeah.
76 E Does your mom cook Chinese food pretty well?
77 C (Um) yeah.
78 E Who else live/3s at your house?
79 C (Um) my grandpa <> and my grandma <> and my dog.
80 E <Uhhuh>.
81 E <Uhhuh>.
82 E And your dog, tell me about your dog?
83 C (Um) he live/3s in (um) my room because he/'s my dog.
84 E Oh.
85 E What does he look like?
86 C Black and blue, I mean black and white.
87 E (Laughing) black and blue.
88 E Black and white.
89 E What kind of dog is it?
90 C I don't know.
91 E A mutt?
92 E Yeah.
93 E What kind/s of thing/s do you and your dog do together?
94 C Play.
95 E Like what?
96 C Play (um um) catch :02 with a frisbee.
97 E Oh yeah?
98 E Hey you know what else I would like to know about?
99 E (What h*) what are the rule/s out there on the playground for (um)sliding?
100 E How can you slide down the hill?
101 C I don't know.
102 C I never done it [EU].
103 E Oh, you never slide down the hill out there?
104 E Why not?
105 C I don't know.
106 C I don't have a sled.
107 E Oh, I thought there were school sled/s.

108 C I don't wanna use them.
109 E Oh, so you don't like to go sled/ing?
110 E You go sled/ing with your mom?
111 C No.
112 ; :03
113 E Or your sister?
114 E No?
115 ; :02
116 E (Um) what/'s your favorite thing to do, (y*) collect baseball card/s?
117 C Play with my dog.
118 E Play with your dog?
119 ; :02
120 E That sound/3s like fun.
121 E You do that everday when you get home?
122 C Yeah.

Analysis of the Data

The conversational language sample was analyzed using SALT and compared to the typically developing seven year olds in the reference database. The data is summarized in the following chart. Both the number of words and utterances per minute were low suggesting a low rate of oral production. The number of different words was four standard deviations from the mean and the total number of words was delayed by three standard deviations. These measures suggest limited semantic diversity or a small vocabulary. Problems with semantic diversity are confirmed by the TTR which is more than two standard deviations above the mean. We can conclude that the child talked very little about each topic that was introduced.

The relatively few conjunctions used during the conversation was another indicator of limited productive language skills. The student did not conjoin utterances very frequently and the syntactic complexity of his conversation was limited. His mean length of utterance was more than three standard deviations below the mean of normal children his age. Further analysis demonstrated that he produced few utterances with errors.

Measurement Category	Student	Mean Seven Year Olds	Standard Deviation
Utterances per Minute	10.58	13.5	2.52
Number Words per Minute	33.56	69.12	16.53
Total Words	320	524	73
Number Different Words	132	188	17
TTR	.52	.45	.05
MLU	3.43	5.76	.79

Language sample analysis confirmed classroom observations of this student. He uses little and unelaborated language with peers and adults. It is also consistent with standardized testing data which suggested an expressive language problem. He does not have the facility to use language in the same ways as his peers and it handicaps him both socially and academically.

Intervention Plan

Therapy is designed to increase the amount of language used by this child. The clinician hypothesized that increased verbal practice would stimulate increased complexity and semantic diversity. Additional attention is directed towards developing strategies to facilitate comprehension and processing of complex, concept loaded, oral directions.

Case Four: Pragmatic Problems
C.A.: 8-3, Grade 2 (Repeated)
Features of the Pragmatic Problems Category
- non-contingent utterances
- pronominal reference errors
- problems with topic maintenance
- new versus old information
- narrative structure

Background Information/Reason for Referral

This student was referred to exceptional education during her kindergarten year after routine kindergarten screening. Her parents had no concerns about her development. No concerns had been expressed by the preschool she attended prior to kindergarten entry that would predict that she would have difficulty in school. Both of her parents received remedial help of an unknown nature in grades K-3. She had one younger sibling, also apparently developing normally. An M-team evaluation completed at this point in time, resulted in a placement offer in a self-contained language program. The parents refused the offer of placement. School concerns persisted through first grade; the following year she was enrolled in a non-public school setting where she repeated first grade. The non-public school felt that she had made minimal progress during that year and recommended retention again. She re-entered the public school to a second grade classroom and was referred by her physician after an EEG showed focal abnormalities.

Results of Standardized Testing

Test of Language Development—Primary:
Picture Vocabulary	SS 8	25 percentile
Oral Vocabulary	SS 6	9 percentile
Grammatic Understanding	SS 6	9 percentile
Grammatic Completion	SS 6	9 percentile
Sentence Imitation	SS 3	1 percentile
Word Discrimination	SS 9	37 percentile

Peabody Picture Vocabulary Test—R:
age equivalent 7-3

WISC—R:
V 75
P 96
FS 84

Scores on tests of math, reading, and writing were all significantly below grade level which was consistent with classroom functioning. She was having more success with rote application of skills and tasks with visual components in both the classroom and during testing. Diagnosticians also noted repeated brief episodes of staring. Standardized language measures were all delayed with respect to her chronological age, but did not help the clinician to discriminate the role that auditory processing deficits and suspected seizure activity played in her poor performance.

Transcript of a Conversational Language Sample

A conversational language sample was elicited and transcribed. The following is an excerpt from the sample:

42	C	And then what mama does is she pick/3s me up by my hand/s and
43		then they toss me on my back.
44	C	And (I d*) I don't like that at all.
45	E	You don't?
46	C	No.
47	E	That/'s sound/3s pretty fun, then you/'d bounce on your bed.
48	C	We have bunkbeds so (I don't) I sleep on the top.
49	C	I don't want to get hit by the bunkbeds.
50	E	No.
51	C	Sometimes I do seat drop/s.
52	E	Yeah.
53	-	1:00
54	C	And what happen/ed is I went to go see the Blueangels at the
55		EEA [CU].
56	E	Mhm.
57	C	And I went to go see some movie/s with my grandma and grandpa.
58	C	And I have some fre* (um)>
59	C	Tomorrow I/'m go/ing over to see (um) Ryanv/z house.
60	C	But (his) I think he>
61	C	I don't know>
62	C	To play.
63	C	And (um) I/'m gonna see (my) my little baby cousin [CU].
64	E	You are?
65	C	Uhhuh.
66	E	At Ryanv/z house?
67	C	No (at) at my counsin/z.
68	E	Oh.
69	C	And I/'m gonna see my AuntLois [CU].
70	:	:04
71	E	Does AuntLois live in Madison?
72	C	No she live/3s in Texas.
73	E	And you/'re gonna do that tomorrow too?
74	C	No (we/'re all gonna we/'re) we have plan/s to do it.

Analysis of the Data

The transcript of the conversational language sample was analyzed using SALT and the results were compared to the typically developing seven and nine year olds in the reference database. As you can see from the data in the chart below, all measures computed by SALT were within one standard deviation of the mean for nine year olds. Errors were noted in her use of bound morphemes which is consistent with her performance on the TOLD-P grammatic understanding, grammatic completion, and sentence imitation subtests. Reading the transcript allowed the clinician to quantify the most striking aspect of her sample—the frequency with which she shifted topics. These frequent abrupt switches in content made conversation with her difficult to follow and sustain.

Measurement Category	Student	Mean Seven Year Olds	Standard Deviation	Mean Nine Year Olds	Standard Deviation
MLU	8.17	5.76	.81	8.8	1.64
TTR	.38	.45	.05	.33	.06
Number Total Words	727	524	74	800	147.7
Number Different Words	220	188	17	204	28.69
Utterances with Mazes	40	25.6	12.4	32.7	10.17

Her parents and teacher confirmed that the sample was typical of her conversational style.

Intervention Plan

A school-wide intervention plan was undertaken. All adults who had frequent conversational exchanges with her used the same cues once a topic had been established and she abruptly switched to another. The adults asked her to recall the topic of conversation and then asked her to establish a relationship between her latest utterance and the topic of conversation. She also received small group therapy focusing on morphology drill, direct practice in turn-taking and topic maintenance in conversation, and strategies to process and remember auditorily presented information. Her family received encouragement to pursue medical management of the suspected seizure disorder.

Case Five: Semantic or Referencing Deficit
C.A.: 4-11, Preschool
Features of the Semantic Deficit Category
- over-generalization, word choice and NP-VP symmetry errors
- abandoned utterances
- redundancy

Background Information/Reason for Referral

This child was referred as a three year old to the school's Early Childhood Program. She received programming from the time of the referral to the present, when a reassessment was initiated to determine the most appropriate programs and services for her as she entered kindergarten. There is a history of learning problems in the family. Her father is described as unable to read or write; her mother received special education classes until she dropped out of school in grade nine.

Results of Standardized Testing

Test of Auditory Comprehension of Language—Revised:

Word Classes and Relations	Below the 1st percentile
Grammatical Morphemes	Below the 1st percentile
Elaborated Sentences	6 percentile
Total Score	Below the 1st percentile

Structural Photographic Expressive Language Test—Preschool:
Below the 1st percentile

Bracken Basic Concept Scale:
Subtests ranged from the 2nd to the 9th percentile
Overall score 5th percentile

Peabody Picture Vocabulary Test—R:
4 percentile

Utah:

Comprehension	SS 2	Below the 1st percentile
Expression	SS 8	25 percentile
Overall	SS 70	2 percentile

Vineland Adaptive Behavior Scales:
Composite SS 58

WPPSI—R:
Composite 1 percentile

This student functioned in the cognitively delayed range on standardized measures of intellectual functioning. There was a significant difference between verbal and performance scores, with verbal being higher. Adaptive and language skills as measured by these standardized tests were consistent with cognitive functioning.

Transcript of a Narrative Language Sample

A narrative language sample was elicited and transcribed. The following is an excerpt from the sample:

```
 1  E  (Let's) let's hear the story of HanselandGretel.
 2  :  :02
 3  C  But the old witch get [EW:got] the stupid kid/s>
 4  C  No.
 5  C  That XX friend.
 6  C  That stuff.
 7  C  And that over there *is SantaClaus.
 8  C  And that *is the witch.
 9  ;  :03
10  C  But you can/'t have a dance (and that stuff and that) all the time
11     [EU] [CU].
12  C  And that X come out.
13  C  But then in the window outside>
14  ;  :06
15  C  But mommy and daddy *are together again.
16  C  And that *is all.
17  C  All *the time.
18  C  But mommy (and) and the kid/s *are together and that stuff.
19  C  And that stuff.
20  ;  :05
21  C  You *are wait/ing now but that stuff>
22  ;  :04
23  C  But all the time and that stuff [EU] [CU].
25 24  C  Mommy and daddy *are together.
26  C  And bunny to a bunny together [EU] [CU].
```

Analysis of the Data

The narrative language sample transcript was analyzed using SALT and compared to the typically developing three year olds and five year olds in the reference database. The

172

three year old comparison was made to allow a comparison of her performance relative to her mental age. As you can see in the chart below, the total number of words and number of different words were delayed when compared to the data from normal five year olds. Neither were significantly low when compared to the three year olds, however, this child may have a limited vocabulary or difficulty finding and using the appropriate word needed to express herself. The mean length of her utterances is also low when compared to five year olds, but again, within the expected performance range for three year olds. The number of utterances with mazes were consistent with the data from five year olds, but significantly higher than the number of mazes produced by normal three year olds.

Measurement Category	Student	Mean Five Year Olds	Standard Deviation*	Mean Three Year Olds	Standard Deviation*
Total Words	351*	440		289	
Different Words	118*	148		103	
MLU	3.67*	5.58		3.59	
Utterances with Mazes	19	14.8		11.8	
Errors					
Word level	5				
Utterance level	12				

* lSD five year olds

Further analysis of the sample showed that she produced many errors at the word and utterance levels. These errors reflected word choice difficulties or unclear reference. The child appeared unable to find the words she needed to encode ideas and events. She frequently used "stuff" and other non-specific words which is consistent with this view of her oral language deficit.

Intervention Plan

Remediation was designed to build vocabulary comprehension and production. Production activities used some repetitive sentence patterns which it was hoped would reduce her need to formulate syntax at the same time she was searching for vocabulary. In addition, classification activities were incorporated into vocabulary practice to aid storage and retrieval.

Case Six: General Delay
C.A.: 4-8, Preschool
Features of the General Delay Category
• decreased number of different words and total number of words
• delayed syntactic development as measured by MLU and other detailed syntactic analyses

Background Information/Reason for Referral

This child was referred to the school district's Early Childhood Program when he was twenty months of age. Concerns were in the areas of cognition, motor skills, social skills, and communication development. He had a medical diagnosis of hypotonia and developmental delay.

He was a full-term baby with no labor, delivery, or neonatal complications. However, all developmental milestones were delayed and there were concerns at about six months of age regarding head size. A CAT scan ruled out hydrocephalus. He is followed by the neurodevelopmental clinic at a local hospital. He is an only child in a single parent family.

Results of Standardized Testing

Preschool Language Scale:
Auditory Comprehension Standard Score 87.5
Verbal Ability Standard Score 83
Language Quotient 84
Chronological Age 4-8

Expressive One Word Picture Vocabulary Test:
Standard Score 84
Chronological Age 4-3

Peabody Picture Vocabulary Test—Revised:
Standard Score 72
Chronological Age 4-8

Developmental Pinpoints, Birth to Six:
Low average to average cognitive skills

Standardized test results profile a student whose language skills are in the low average range with poorer skills in comprehension of single word vocabulary. For the most part, his performance on measures of language ability are consistent with estimates of his cognitive ability and are about one standard deviation from the mean.

Transcript of a Conversational Language Sample

A conversational language sample was elicited and transcribed. The following is an excerpt from the transcript:

```
 3  E  Oh, you know what, I have Mr. Potatohead here too.
 4  E  Do you like Mr. Potatohead?
 5  C  Yeah.
 6  E  Wanna see what he/'s do/ing?
 7  E  <Sit down>.
 8  C  <Ye*>>
 9  E  Here/'s Mr. Potatohead.
10  C  What you make [EU]?
11  E  We can make Mr. Potatohead.
12  E  I/'ll get out all the piece/s and you can <see (what) what he>
13  C  <(Um um)> XX.
14  C  He does/n't have a face.
15  E  He does/n't have a face you/'re right.
16  :  :03
17  C  Gonna make [EU].
18  E  What should we make?
19  E  You know what, I think he need/3s to stand up first.
20  E  What do you think?
21  C  Mhm.
22  E  But you need to sit down.
23  E  That/'s a boy.
24  ;  :02
```

25 E Ok <here/'s Mr. Potat*>

26 C <Oh>.

27 E (What di*) What did I do?

28 E What did <I do>?

29 C <The> face.

30 C <No> I don't <wanna>.

31 E (<K*>) <Alright> you tell me what you would like.

32 C (Um) a pink [EU].

33 E What are these pink thing/s?

34 C (Um) eye/s.

35 E They/'re not eye/s, but [p].

36 C Nose.

37 E Not nose/s.

38 : :03

39 C Ear/s.

40 E Ear/s, where do ear/s go?

41 C Right <here>.

42 E <Ok> good.

43 E Now Mr. Potatohead can hear.

44 C That/'s hat [EU].

45 E Is that where his hat go/3s?

46 C Yes.

47 E Ok you tell me what else you would like.

48 E I/'m gonna (p*) put all the thing/s out right here.

49 E What else would you like to put on Mr. Potatohead today?

50 C Hat.

51 : :04

52 E There/'s his hat.

Analysis of the Data

The language sample transcript was analyzed using SALT and the child's performance was compared to the reference database of typically developing five year olds. Significant data is summarized in the chart below. As you can see, his mean length of utterance (MLU) of 1.97 morphemes is approximately three standard deviations below the mean of children his age. His performance places him in Brown's Late Stage I with an age range of 18-31 months. His spontaneous language production is characterized by little complexity and by many syntactic and grammatical errors. Both the total number of words used and the number of different words used are significantly delayed as well, and reflect difficulty in semantics. He was observed using gestures and other non-verbal means of communication as well as incorrectly labelling familiar things in his environment during the language sample.

Measurement Category	Student	Mean Five Year Olds	Standard Deviation
MLU	1.97	5.69	1.03
TTR	.57	.44	.05
Number Total Words	197	517	91
Number Different Words	69	175	27

Although a semantic delay might have been suspected from the standardized test information, the other characteristics of a general delay across areas of language development are only described when language sample analysis is used as a diagnostic strategy.

Intervention Plan

The language sample analysis helps to plan appropriate therapy and classroom based intervention activities. This child needs to expand his utterances to include more complexity and greater length. He needs to learn the labels for common objects and actions in his environment and use those words to express ideas and observations about his world more completely and effectively. His clinician and early childhood classroom teacher are using meaningful, familiar contexts like snack and play time to foster general language development. In this way, a variety of language structures and vocabulary can be practiced in a functional setting.

Case Seven: Dismissal; LSA documented no need for continued services
C.A.: 15-7, Grade 9

Background Information/Reason for Referral

This student was first identified as handicapped and in need of exceptional education in the spring of his first grade year. He received speech and language and learning disabilities support from then until the current evaluation. The amount of support has gradually decreased and the time spent in regular education classes has increased.

The last reassessment completed in grade six documented a need for continued language intervention using a Loban analysis of a narrative language sample. At that time, the student used an average of 6.56 words per communication unit, with .20 dependent clauses per communication unit. This performance is significantly delayed for sixth grade students in Loban's sample. Maze information from the same sample was unremarkable. The student frequently reported that assessment tasks requiring verbal fluency were too difficult, and he did appear to struggle with verbal expression. Measures of comprehension were all in the average range. At the beginning of his ninth grade year, the student was promised that he could be dismissed from therapy if he worked hard and applied what he was learning to academic classes. He immediately began to focus on increasing sentence length in both writing and talking. He began to increase both the amount and variety of conjunctions that he could use correctly in therapy and worked at applying conjunction use in assigned homework.

Results of Standardized Testing

All productive language measures computed by SALT were within normal limits at the time of the last assessment. As a result, no standardized tests were readministered at this time.

Transcript of a Narrative Language Sample

A narrative language sample was elicited and transcribed. The following is an excerpt from the transcript:

```
1  C  (But and the* there) first this like cop came over (to check on) to
2     ask them if they had any way to check if their house was safe.
3  C  And the cop had kept on ask/ing is your father here?
4  C  (And y*) they were like nope.
5  C  And he kept on ask/ing because he could never find out who/z
6     father own/ed the house.
7  C  And then a pizza guy came and drop/ed off the pizza/s.
8  C  He wait/ed there for a long time try/ing to find out (the) who was
9     the real guy there.
```

176

10 C (Because they) well they all came over because they were gonna
11   go over to Paris.
12 C (And then) well that/'s where the people (that) were visit/ing.
13 C Then they were all gonna go back over to Paris.
14 C And :03 then well the one that was about four, (he um) he was like
15   not ready [EW: already] pack/ed and he kept on ask/ing people (how
16   he got) how you pack/ed.
17 C Everybody kept on call/ing him baby and all that because he
18   could/n't do it.
19 C And then later, after all that, they they went to go.
20 C They ate supper :03 and he start/ed to yell at his older brother.

Analysis of the Data

The narrative language sample transcript was analyzed using SALT and the results were compared to the typically developing 13 year olds in the reference database. All of the language measures computed by SALT were in the average range when compared to the 13-year-old speakers. Sentence length was well above average, and the clinician felt that accounted for the below average performance reflected in "utterances per minute."

Measurement Category	Student	Mean 13 Year Olds	Standard Deviation
MLU	13.21	9.32	1.49
TTR	.30	.36	.03
Number Total Words	1190.00	842.11	27.43
Number Different Word Roots	274.00	237.00	132.43
Number Words per Minute	127.14	130.59	24.91
Number Utterances per Minute	11.38	16.33	3.61
Mazes	40.00	37.44	11.42
Overlaps	8.65	7.56	5.67
Number Pauses	4.00	2.11	3.56
Number Pauses	2.00	2.63	4.00

Further analysis indicated that 30 of the 40 mazes were one word in length. The student gave specific information during the narrative, detailing the relationships between characters and events. He used intonation and facial expressions that contributed to the listener's perception of communicative competency. Academic grades also reflected improvement in language ability and motivation.

Dialectical and Bilingual Considerations[*]

Most regional and ethnic dialects differ only slightly from the standard or are used by a limited number of individuals. Three ethnic dialects, however, represent rather large segments of the U.S. population and have some very important differences with Standard American English. These dialects are Black English, Hispanic English, and Asian English. Black English is used primarily by working-class Blacks in the northern U.S. and rural Blacks in the south. Not every African-American uses Black English and not everyone who uses it is an African-American.

Hispanic English and Asian English are probably misnomers. Hispanic English, as used here, is a composite of the English used by many bilingual speakers who learned English as a second language. Individual variations represent the age of learning and level of mastery, the Spanish dialect used, socioeconomic status, and where the person lives in the United States. Asian English is also a composite, but of bilingual Asian speakers who learned English as a second language. As such, Asian English probably does not exist except to simplify our discussion. Asians speak many different languages, and each has a different effect on the learning of English. In addition to the original language learned, other individual differences may reflect factors the same as those of Hispanic English.

Each dialect is discussed in some detail. Where possible, information has been reduced to tables to aid presentation. Each dialect is compared with Standard American English, an idealized norm uninfluenced by the dialectal differences each person possesses.

Black English

Black English reflects the complex racial and economic history of the United States and the migration of African-Americans from the rural south to the urban north after World War II. Regional differences exist to some degree. The major variations between Standard American English and Black English in phonology, syntax, and morphology and in pragmatics and nonlinguistic features are presented in Tables B.1 and B.2.

---

[*] Reprinted with the permission of Merrill, an imprint of MacMillan Publishing Company, from *Language Disorders: A Functional Approach to Assessment and Intervention* by Robert E. Owens. ©1991 by MacMillan Publishing Company.

Table B.1

Phonemic contrasts between Black English and Standard American English

Standard American English Phonemes	Position in Word		
	Initial	Medial	Final[*]
/p/		Unaspirated /p/	Unaspirated /p/
/n/			Reliance on preceding nazalized vowel
/w/	Omitted in specific words (*I'as, too!*)		
/b/		Unreleased /b/	Unreleased /b/
/g/		Unreleased /g/	Unreleased /g/
/k/		Unaspirated /k/	Unaspirated /k/
/d/	Omitted in specific words (*I'on't know*)	Unreleased /d/	Unreleased /d/
/ŋ/		/n/	/n/
/t/		Unaspirated /t/	Unaspirated /t/
/l/		Omitted before labial consonants (*help-hep*)	"uh" following a vowel (*Bill-Biuh*)
/r/		Omitted or /ə/	Omitted or prolonged vowel or glide
/θ/	Unaspirated /t/ or /f/	Unaspirated /t/ or /f/ between vowels	Unaspirated /t/ or /f/ (*bath-baf*)
/v/	Sometimes /b/	/b/ before /m/ and /n/	Sometimes /b/
/ð/	/d/	/d/ or /v/ between vowels	/d/, /v/, /f/
/z/		Omitted or replaced by /d/ before nasal sound (*wasn't-wud'n*)	

Blends

/str/ becomes /skr/
/ʃr/ becomes /str/
/θr/ becomes /θ/
/pr/ becomes /p/
/br/ becomes /b/
/kr/ becomes /k/
/gr/ becomes /g/

Final Consonant Clusters (second consonant omitted when these clusters occur at the end of a word)

/sk/	/nd/	/sp/
/ft/	/ld/	/d₃ d/
/st/	/sd/	/nt/

---

[*] Note weakening of final consonants.

Sources: Data drawn from Fasold and Wolfram (1970); Labov (1972); F. Weiner and Lewnau (1979); R. Williams and Wolfram (1977).

Table B.2

Grammatical contrasts between Black English and Standard American English

Black English Grammatical Structure	Standard American English Grammatical Structure
Possessive -'s	
Nonobligatory where word position expresses possession.	Obligatory regardless of position.
Get *mother* coat.	Get mother's coat.
It be mother's.	It's mother's.
Plural -s	
Nonobligatory with numerical quantifier.	Obligatory regardless of numerical quantifier.
He got ten *dollar*.	He has ten dollars.
Look at the cats.	Look at the cats.
Regular past -ed	
Nonobligatory; reduced as consonant cluster.	Obligatory.
Yesterday, I *walk* to school.	Yesterday, I walked to school.
Irregular past	
Case by case, some verbs inflected, others not.	All irregular verbs inflected.
I *see* him last week.	I *saw* him last week.
Regular present tense third person singular -s	
Nonobligatory.	Obligatory.
She *eat* too much.	She eats too much.
Irregular present tense third person singular -s	
Nonobligatory.	Obligatory.
He *do* my job.	He *does* my job.
Indefinite an	
Use of indefinite *a*.	Use of *an* before nouns beginning with a vowel.
He ride in *a* airplane.	He rode in *an* airplane.
Pronouns	
Pronominal apposition: pronoun immediately follows noun.	Pronoun used elsewhere in sentence or in other sentence: not in apposition.
Momma *she* mad. She . . .	Momma is mad. *She* . . .

(continued)

Table B.2 *(continued)*

Black English Grammatical Structure	Standard American English Grammatical Structure
Future tense	
More frequent use of *be going to* (gonna).	More frequent use of *will*.
I *be going to* dance tonight.	I *will* dance tonight.
I *gonna* dance tonight.	I *am going to* dance tonight.
Omit *will* preceding *be*.	Obligatory use of *will*.
I *be* home later.	I *will* (I'll) *be* home later.
Negation	
Triple negative.	Absence of triple negative.
Nobody don't never like me.	*No* one ever likes me.
Use of *ain't*.	*Ain't* is unacceptable form.
I *ain't* going.	I'm *not* going.
Modals	
Double modals for such forms as might, *could*, and *should*.	Single modal use.
I *might could* go.	I *might be able to* go.
Questions	
Same form for direct and indirect.	Different forms for direct and indirect.
What *is it*?	What *is* it?
Do you know what *it is*?	Do you know what *it is*?
Relative pronouns	
Nonobligatory in most cases.	Nonobligatory with *that* only.
He the one stole it.	He's the one *who* stole it.
It the one you like.	It's the one (that) you like.
Conditional *if*	
Use of *do* for conditional *if*.	Use of *if*.
I ask *did* she go.	I asked *if* she went.
Perfect construction	
Been used for action in the distant past: He *been* gone.	*Been* not used: He left a long time ago.
Copula	
Nonobligatory when contractible: He sick.	Obligatory in contractible and uncontractible forms: He's sick.
Habitual or general state	
Marked with uninflected *be*.	Nonuse of *be*; verb inflected.
She *be* workin'.	She's *working* now.

Sources: Data drawn from Baratz (1969), Fasold and Wolfram (1970), Williams and Wolfram (1977).

Hispanic English

Bilingual speakers may move back and forth between both languages in a process called *code switching*. The amount of code switching depends on the speaker's mastery of the two languages and on the audience being addressed. Naturally, a large amount of code switching makes the speaker's English incomprehensible to the monolingual American English listener.

Most characteristics of Hispanic English reflect interference points or points where the two languages differ, thus making learning somewhat more difficult. For example, the Hispanic English speaker may continue to use the Spanish possessive form in which the owner is preceded by the entity owned, as in "the dress of Mary." The major variations between Standard American English and Hispanic English in phonology, syntax, and morphology and in pragmatics and nonlinguistic features are presented in Tables B.4 and B.5.

Table B.4
Phonemic contrasts between Hispanic English and Standard American English

Standard American English Phonemes	Position in Word		
	Initial	Medial	Final*
/p/	Unaspirated /p/		Omitted or weakened
/m/			Omitted
/w/	/hu/		Omitted
/b/			Omitted, distorted, or /p/
/g/			Omitted, distorted, or /k/
/k/	Unaspirated or /g/		Omitted, distorted, or /g/
/f/			Omitted
/d/		Dentalized	Omitted, distorted, or /t/
/ŋ/	/n/	/d/	/n/ (*sing-sin*)
/j/	/dʒ/		
/t/			Omitted
/ʃ/	/tʃ/	/s/, /tʃ/	/tʃ/ (*wish-which*)
/tʃ/	/ʃ/ (*chair-share*)	/ʃ/	/ʃ/ (*watch-wash*)
/r/	Distorted	Distorted	Distorted
/dʒ/	/d/	/j/	/ʃ/
/θ/	/t/, /s/ (*thin-tin, sin*)	Omitted	/ʃ/, /t/ or /s/
/v/	/b/ (*vat-bat*)	/b/	Distorted
/z/	/s/ (*zip-sip*)	/s/ (*razor-racer*)	/s/
/ð/	/d/ (*then-den*)	/d/, /θ/, /v/ (*lather-ladder*)	/d/

Blends

/skw/ becomes /eskw/*
/sl/   becomes /esl/*
/st/   becomes /est/*

Vowels

/ɪ/ becomes /i/ (*bit-beet*)

---

* Separates cluster into two syllables.

Sources: Data drawn from Sawyer (1973); F. Weiner and Lewnau (1979); F. Williams, Cairns, and Cairns (1971).

Table B.5
Grammatical contrasts between Hispanic English and Standard American English

Hispanic English Grammatical Structure	Standard American English Grammatical Structure
Possessive -'s	
Use postnoun modifier.	Postnoun modifier used only rarely.
This is the homework *of my brother*.	This is my brother's homework.
Article used with body parts.	Possessive pronoun used with body parts.
I cut *the* finger.	I cut *my* finger.
Plural -s	
Nonobligatory.	Obligatory, excluding exceptions.
The *girl* are playing.	The *girls* are playing.
The *sheep* are playing.	The *sheep* are playing.
Regular past -ed	
Nonobligatory; especially when understood.	Obligatory.
I *talk* to her yesterday.	I *talked* to her yesterday.
Regular third person singular present tense -s	
Nonobligatory.	Obligatory.
She *eat* too much.	She *eats* too much.
Articles	
Often omitted.	Usually obligatory.
I am going to store.	I am going to *the* store.
I am going to school.	I am going to school.
Subject pronouns	
Omitted when subject has been identified in the previous sentence.	Obligatory.
Father is happy. Bought a new car.	Father is happy. *He* bought a new car.
Future tense	
Use *go + to*.	Use *be + going to*.
I *go to* dance.	I *am going to* the dance.
Negation	
Use *no* before the verb.	Use *not* (preceded by auxiliary verb where appropriate).
She *no* eat candy.	She does *not* eat candy.

(continued)

Table B.5 *(continued)*

Hispanic English Grammatical Structure	Standard American English Grammatical Structure
Question	
Intonation; no noun-verb inversion.	Noun-verb inversion usually.
Maria is going?	*Is Maria* going?
Copula	
Occasional use of *have*.	Use of *be*.
I *have* ten years.	I *am* ten years old.
Negative imperatives	
No used for *don't*.	*Don't* used.
No throw stones.	*Don't* throw stones.
***Do* insertion**	
Nonobligatory in questions.	Obligatory when no auxiliary verb.
You like ice cream?	*Do* you like ice cream?
Comparatives	
More frequent use of longer form (more).	More frequent use of shorter *-er*.
He is *more* tall.	He is *taller*.

Sources: Data drawn from Davis (1972), Taylor (1986).

Asian English

Chinese culture and language have for centuries influenced all other Asian cultures and languages. Other cultures, such as that of the Indian subcontinent, have influenced nearby Asian neighbors. Colonial occupation, especially by the French in Indochina, has also influenced the culture and language of the affected region.

The most widely used languages, Chinese, Filipino, Japanese, Khmer, Korean, Laotian, and Vietnamese, represent only a portion of the languages of the area. Each language contains many dialects and has distinct linguistic features. It is, therefore, impossible to speak of an Asian English dialect. Instead, we shall attempt to describe the major overall differences between Asian English and Standard American English. These major differences in phonology, syntax, and morphology and pragmatics and nonlinguistic features are listed in Tables. B.7 and B.8.

Table B.7
Phonemic contrasts between Asian English and Standard American English

Standard American English Phonemes	Position in Word		
	Initial	Medial	Final
/p/	/b/****	/b/****	Omission
/s/	Distortion*	Distortion*	Omission
/z/	/s/**	/s/**	Omission
/t/	Distortion*	Distortion*	Omission
/tʃ/	/ʃ/****	/ʃ/****	Omission
/ʃ/	/s/**	/s/**	Omission
/r/, /l/	Confusion***	Confusion***	Omission
/θ/	/s/	/s/	Omission
/dz/	/d/ or /z/****	/d/ or /z/****	Omission
/v/	/f/***	/f/***	Omission
	/w/**	/w/**	Omission
/ð/	/z/*	/z/*	Omission
	/d/****	/d/****	Omission

Blends

    Addition of // between consonants***
    Omission of final consonant clusters****

Vowels

    Shortening or lengthening of vowels (*seat-sit, it-eat**)
    Difficulty with /I/, /ɔ/, and /æ/, and substitution of /e/ for /æ/**
    Difficulty with /I/, /æ/, /U/, and /ə/****

*	Mandarin dialect of Chinese only
**	Cantonese dialect of Chinese only
***	Mandarin, Cantonese, and Japanese
****	Vietnamese only

Source: Adapted from Cheng, L. (June 1987). Cross-cultural and linguistic considerations in working with Asian populations. *Asha, 29*(6), p. 33-38.

Table B.8
Grammatical contrasts between Asian English and Standard American English

Asian English Grammatical Structure	Standard American English Grammatical Structure
Plural -s	
Not used with numerical adjective: *three cat*	Used regardless of numerical adjective: *three cats*
Used with irregular plural: *three sheeps*	Not used with irregular plural: *three sheep*
Auxiliaries *to be* and *to do*	
Omission: *I going home. She not want eat.*	Obligatory and inflected in the present progressive form: *I am going home. She does not want to eat.*
Uninflected: *I is going. She do not want eat.*	
Verb *have*	
Omission: *You been here.*	Obligatory and inflected: *You have been here. He has one.*
Uninflected: *He have one.*	
Past tense -ed	
Omission: *He talk yesterday.*	Obligatory, nonovergeneralization, and single-marking: *He talked yesterday. I ate yesterday. She didn't eat.*
Overgeneralization: *I eated yesterday.*	
Double-marking: *She didn't ate.*	
Interrogative	
Nonreversal: *You ate late?*	Reversal and obligatory auxiliary: *Are you late? Do you like ice cream?*
Omitted auxiliary: *You like ice cream?*	
Perfect marker	
Omission: *I have write letter.*	Obligatory: *I have written a letter.*
Verb-noun agreement	
Nonagreement: *He go to school. You goes to school.*	Agreement: *He goes to school. You go to school.*
Article	
Omission: *Please give gift.*	Obligatory with certain nouns: *Please give the gift. She went to school.*
Overgeneralization: *She go the school.*	
Preposition	
Misuse: *I am in home.*	Obligatory specific use: *I am at home. He goes by bus.*
Omission: *He go bus.*	

(continued)

Table B.8 *(continued)*

Asian English Grammatical Structure	Standard American English Grammatical Structure
Pronoun	
Subjective/objective confusion: *Him go quickly.*	Subjective/objective distinction: *He gave it to her.*
Possessive confusion: *It him book.*	Possessive distinction: *It's his book.*
Demonstrative	
Confusion: *I like those horse.*	Singular/plural distinction: *I like that horse.*
Conjunction	
Omission: *You I go together.*	Obligatory use between last two items in a series: *You and I are going together.* *Mary, John, and Carol went.*
Negation	
Double-marking: *I didn't see nobody.*	Single obligatory marking: *I didn't see anybody.* *He didn't come.*
Simplified form: *He no come.*	
Word order	
Adjective following noun (Vietnamese): *clothes new.*	Most noun modifiers precede noun: *new clothes.*
Possessive following noun (Vietnamese): *dress her.*	Possessive precedes noun: *her dress.*
Omission of object with transitive verb: *I want.*	Use of direct object with most transitive verbs: *I want it.*

Source: Adapted from Cheng, L. (June 1987). Cross-cultural and linguistic considerations in working with Asian populations. *Asha, 29*(6), p. 33-38.